ASIAN RECIPES

MOUTH-WATERING AND DELICIOUS RECIPES TO SURPRISE YOUR FAMILY

PETER GOLDMAN

Table of Contents

3

Sweet and Sour Carp

Serves 4

1 large carp or similar fish
300 g/11 oz/¬œ cup cornflour (cornstarch)
250 ml/8 fl oz/1 cup vegetable oil
30 ml/2 tbsp soy sauce
5 ml/1 tsp salt
150 g/5 oz/heaped ¬Ω cup sugar
75 ml/5 tbsp wine vinegar
15 ml/1 tbsp rice wine or dry sherry
3 spring onions (scallions), finely chopped
1 slice ginger root, finely chopped
250 ml/8 fl oz/1 cup boiling water

Clean and scale the fish and soak it for several hours in cold water. Drain and pat dry then score each side several times. Reserve 30 ml/2 tbsp of cornflour then gradually mix enough water into the remaining cornflour to make a stiff batter. Coat the fish in the batter. Heat the oil until very hot and deep-fry the fish until crisp on the outside then turn down the heat and continue to fry until the fish is tender. Meanwhile, mix together the remaining cornflour, the soy sauce, salt, sugar, wine vinegar, wine or sherry, spring onions and ginger. When the fish is cooked, transfer it to a warm serving plate. Add the sauce mixture and the water to the oil and bring to the boil, stirring well until the sauce thickens. Pour over the fish and serve immediately.

Carp with Tofu

Serves 4

1 carp

60 ml/4 tbsp groundnut (peanut) oil

225 g/8 oz tofu, cubed

2 spring onions (scallions), finely chopped

1 clove garlic, finely chopped

2 slices ginger root, finely chopped

15 ml/1 tbsp chilli sauce

30 ml/2 tbsp soy sauce

500 ml/16 fl oz/2 cups stock

30 ml/2 tbsp rice wine or dry sherry

15 ml/1 tbsp cornflour (cornstarch)

30 ml/2 tbsp water

Trim, scale and clean the fish and score 3 lines diagonally on each side. Heat the oil and fry the tofu gently until golden brown. Remove from the pan and drain well. Add the fish to the pan and fry until golden brown then remove from the pan. Pour off all but 15 ml/1 tbsp of oil then stir-fry the spring onions, garlic and ginger for 30 seconds. Add the chilli sauce, soy sauce, stock and wine and bring to the boil. Carefully add the fish to the pan with the tofu and simmer, uncovered, for about 10 minutes until the fish is cooked and the sauce reduced. Transfer the fish to a warmed serving plate and spoon the tofu on top. Blend the cornflour and water to a paste, stir it into the sauce and simmer, stirring, until the sauce thickens slightly. Spoon over the fish and serve at once.

Almond Fish Rolls

Serves 4

100 g/4 oz/1 cup almonds

450 g/1 lb cod fillets

4 slices smoked ham

1 spring onion (scallion), minced

1 slice ginger root, minced

5 ml/1 tsp cornflour (cornstarch)

5 ml/1 tsp sugar

2.5 ml/¬Ω tsp salt

15 ml/1 tbsp soy sauce

15 ml/1 tbsp rice wine or dry sherry

1 egg, lightly beaten

oil for deep-frying

1 lemon, cut into wedges

Blanch the almonds in boiling water for 5 minutes then drain and mince. Cut the fish into 9 cm/3¬Ω in squares and the ham into 5 cm/2 in squares. Mix the spring onion, ginger, cornflour, sugar, salt, soy sauce, wine or sherry and egg. Dip the fish in the mixture then lay the fish on a work surface. Coat the top with almonds then lay a slice of ham on top. Roll up the fish and tie with cook, Heat the oil and fry the fish rolls for a few minutes until golden brown. Drain on kitchen paper and serve with lemon.

Cod with Bamboo Shoots

Serves 4

4 dried Chinese mushrooms

900 g/2 lb cod fillets, cubed

30 ml/2 tbsp cornflour (cornstarch)

oil for deep-frying

30 ml/2 tbsp groundnut (peanut) oil

1 spring onion (scallion), sliced

1 slice ginger root, minced

salt

100 g/4 oz bamboo shoots, sliced

120 ml/4 fl oz/¬Ω cup fish stock

15 ml/1 tbsp soy sauce

45 ml/3 tbsp water

Soak the mushrooms in warm water for 30 minutes then drain.
Discard the stalks and slice the caps. Dust the fish with half the

cornflour. Heat the oil and deep-fry the fish until golden brown. Drain on kitchen paper and keep warm.

Meanwhile, heat the oil and fry the spring onion, ginger and salt until lightly browned. Add the bamboo shoots and stir-fry for 3 minutes. Add the stock and soy sauce, bring to the boil and simmer for 3 minutes. Mix the remaining cornflour to a paste with the water, stir into the pan and simmer, stirring, until the sauce thickens. Pour over the fish and serve at once.

Fish with Bean Sprouts

Serves 4

450 g/1 lb bean sprouts

45 ml/3 tbsp groundnut (peanut) oil

5 ml/1 tsp salt

3 slices ginger root, minced

450 g/1 lb fish fillets, sliced

4 spring onions (scallions), sliced

15 ml/1 tbsp soy sauce

60 ml/4 tbsp fish stock

10 ml/2 tsp cornflour (cornstarch)

15 ml/1 tbsp water

Blanch the bean sprouts in boiling water for 4 minutes then drain well. Heat half the oil and fry the salt and ginger for 1 minute. Add the fish and fry until lightly browned then remove it from the pan. Heat the remaining oil and fry the spring onions for 1 minute. Add the soy sauce and stock and bring to the boil. Return the fish to the pan, cover and simmer for 2 minutes until the fish is cooked. Mix the cornflour and water to a paste, stir into the pan and simmer, stirring, until the sauce clears and thickens.

Fish Fillets in Brown Sauce

Serves 4

450 g/1 lb cod fillets, thickly sliced

30 ml/2 tbsp rice wine or dry sherry

30 ml/2 tbsp soy sauce

3 spring onions (scallions), finely chopped

1 slice ginger root, finely chopped

5 ml/1 tsp salt

5 ml/1 tsp sesame oil

30 ml/2 tbsp cornflour (cornstarch)

3 eggs, beaten

90 ml/6 tbsp groundnut (peanut) oil

90 ml/6 tbsp fish stock

Place the fish fillets in a bowl. Mix together the wine or sherry, soy sauce, spring onions, ginger, salt and sesame oil, pour over the fish, cover and leave to marinate for 30 minutes. Remove the fish from the marinade and toss in the cornflour then dip in the beaten egg. Heat the oil and fry the fish until golden brown on the outside. Pour off the oil and stir in the stock and any remaining marinade. Bring to the boil and simmer gently for about 5 minutes until the fish is cooked.

Chinese Fish Cakes

Serves 4

450 g/1 lb minced (ground) cod

2 spring onions (scallions), finely chopped

1 clove garlic, crushed

5 ml/1 tsp salt

5 ml/1 tsp sugar

5 ml/1 tsp soy sauce

45 ml/3 tbsp vegetable oil

15 ml/1 tbsp cornflour (cornstarch)

Mix together the cod, spring onions, garlic, salt, sugar, soy sauce and 10 ml/2 tsp of oil. Knead together thoroughly, sprinkling with a little cornflour from time to time until the mixture is soft and elastic. Shape into 4 fish cakes. Heat the oil and fry the fish cakes for about 10 minutes until golden, pressing them flat as they cook. Serve hot or cold.

Crispy-Fried Fish

Serves 4

450 g/1 lb fish fillets, cut into strips

30 ml/2 tbsp rice wine or dry sherry

salt and freshly ground pepper

45 ml/3 tbsp cornflour (cornstarch)

1 egg white, lightly beaten

oil for deep-frying

Toss the fish in the wine or sherry and season with salt and pepper. Dust lightly with cornflour. Beat the remaining cornflour into the egg white until stiff then dip the fish in the batter. Heat the oil and deep-fry the fish strips for a few minutes until golden brown.

Deep-Fried Cod

Serves 4

900 g/2 lb cod fillets, cubed

salt and freshly ground pepper

2 eggs, beaten

100 g/4 oz/1 cup plain (all-purpose) flour

oil for deep-frying

1 lemon, cut into wedges

Season the cod with salt and pepper. Beat the eggs and flour to a batter and season with salt. Dip the fish in the batter. Heat the oil and deep-fry the fish for a few minutes until golden brown and cooked through. Drain on kitchen paper and serve with lemon wedges.

Five-Spice Fish

Serves 4

4 cod fillets

5 ml/1 tsp five-spice powder

5 ml/1 tsp salt

30 ml/2 tbsp groundnut (peanut) oil

2 cloves garlic, crushed

2.5 ml/1 in root ginger, minced

30 ml/2 tbsp rice wine or dry sherry

15 ml/1 tbsp soy sauce

few drops of sesame oil

Rub the fish with the five-spice powder and salt. Heat the oil and fry the fish until lightly browned on both sides. Remove from the pan and add the remaining ingredients. Heat through, stirring, then return the fish to the pan and reheat gently before serving.

Fragrant Fish Sticks

Serves 4

30 ml/2 tbsp rice wine or dry sherry

1 spring onion (scallion), finely chopped

2 eggs, beaten

10 ml/2 tsp curry powder

5 ml/1 tsp salt

450 g/1 lb white fish fillets, cut into strips

100 g/4 oz breadcrumbs

oil for deep-frying

Mix together the wine or sherry, spring onion, eggs, curry powder and salt. Dip the fish into the mixture so that the pieces are evenly coated then press them into the breadcrumbs. Heat the oil and deep-fry the fish for a few minutes until crisp and golden brown. Drain well and serve immediately.

Fish with Gherkins

Serves 4

4 white fish fillets

75 g/3 oz small gherkins

2 spring onions (scallions)

2 slices ginger root

30 ml/2 tbsp water

5 ml/1 tsp groundnut (peanut) oil

2.5 ml/¬Ω tsp salt

2.5 ml/¬Ω tsp rice wine or dry sherry

Place the fish on a heatproof plate and sprinkle with the remaining ingredients. Place on a rack in a steamer, cover and steam for about 15 minutes over boiling water until the fish is tender. Transfer to a warmed serving plate, discard the ginger and spring onions and serve.

Ginger-Spiced Cod

Serves 4

225 g/8 oz tomato purée (paste)

30 ml/2 tbsp rice wine or dry sherry

15 ml/1 tbsp grated ginger root

15 ml/1 tbsp chilli sauce

15 ml/1 tbsp water

15 ml/1 tbsp soy sauce

10 ml/2 tsp sugar

3 cloves garlic, crushed

100 g/4 oz/1 cup plain (all-purpose) flour

75 ml/5 tbsp cornflour (cornstarch)

175 ml/6 fl oz/¾ cup water

1 egg white

2.5 ml/½ tsp salt

oil for deep-frying

450 g/1 lb cod fillets, skinned and cubed

To make the sauce, mix together the tomato purée, wine or sherry, ginger, chilli sauce, water, soy sauce, sugar and garlic. Bring to the boil then simmer, stirring, for 4 minutes.

Beat together the flour, cornflour, water, egg white and salt until smooth. Heat the oil. Dip the fish pieces in the batter and fry for about 5 minutes until cooked through and golden brown. Drain on kitchen paper. Drain off all the oil and return the fish and sauce to the pan. Reheat gently for about 3 minutes until the fish is completely coated in sauce.

Cod with Mandarin Sauce

Serves 4

675 g/1¬Ω lb cod fillets, cut into strips

30 ml/2 tbsp cornflour (cornstarch)

60 ml/4 tbsp groundnut (peanut) oil

1 spring onion (scallion), chopped

2 cloves garlic, crushed

1 slice ginger root, minced

100 g/4 oz mushrooms, sliced

50 g/2 oz bamboo shoots, cut into strips

120 ml/4 fl oz/¬Ω cup soy sauce

30 ml/2 tbsp rice wine or dry sherry

15 ml/1 tbsp brown sugar

5 ml/1 tsp salt

250 ml/8 fl oz/1 cup chicken stock

Dip the fish in the cornflour until lightly coated. Heat the oil and fry the fish until golden brown on both sides. Remove it from the pan. Add the spring onion, garlic and ginger and stir-fry until lightly browned. Add the mushrooms and bamboo shoots and stir-fry for 2 minutes. Add the remaining ingredients and bring to the boil, stirring. Return the fish to the pan, cover and simmer for 20 minutes.

Fish with Pineapple

Serves 4

450 g/1 lb fish fillets

2 spring onions (scallions), minced

30 ml/2 tbsp soy sauce

15 ml/1 tbsp rice wine or dry sherry

2.5 ml/¬Ω tsp salt

2 eggs, lightly beaten

15 ml/1 tbsp cornflour (cornstarch)

45 ml/3 tbsp groundnut (peanut) oil

225 g/8 oz canned pineapple chunks in juice

Cut the fish into 2.5 cm/1 in strips against the grain and place in a bowl. Add the spring onions, soy sauce, wine or sherry and salt, toss well and leave to stand for 30 minutes. Drain the fish, discarding the marinade. Beat the eggs and cornflour to a batter and dip the fish in the batter to coat, draining off any excess. Heat the oil and fry the fish until lightly browned on both sides. Reduce the heat and continue to cook until tender. Meanwhile, mix 60 ml/4 tbsp of the pineapple juice with any remaining batter and the pineapple chunks. Place in a pan over a gentle heat and simmer until heated through, stirring continuously. Arrange the cooked fish on a warmed serving plate and pour over the sauce to serve.

Fish Rolls with Pork

Serves 4

450 g/1 lb fish fillets

100 g/4 oz cooked pork, minced (ground)

30 ml/2 tbsp rice wine or dry sherry

15 ml/1 tbsp sugar

oil for deep-frying

120 ml/4 fl oz/¬Ω cup fish stock

3 spring onions (scallions), minced

1 slice ginger root, minced

15 ml/1 tbsp soy sauce

15 ml/1 tbsp cornflour (cornstarch)

45 ml/3 tbsp water

Cut the fish into 9 cm/3¬Ω in squares. Mix the pork with the wine or sherry and half the sugar, spread over the fish squares, roll them up and secure with string. Heat the oil and deep-fry the fish until golden brown. Drain on kitchen paper. Meanwhile, heat the stock and add the spring onions, ginger, soy sauce and remaining sugar. Bring to the boil and simmer for 4 minutes. Mix the cornflour and water to a paste, stir into the pan and simmer, stirring, until the sauce clears and thickens. Pour over the fish and serve at once.

Fish in Rice Wine

Serves 4

400 ml/14 fl oz/1¬œ cups rice wine or dry sherry

120 ml/4 fl oz/¬Ω cup water

30 ml/2 tbsp soy sauce

5 ml/1 tsp sugar

salt and freshly ground pepper

10 ml/2 tsp cornflour (cornstarch)

15 ml/1 tbsp water

450 g/1 lb cod fillets

5 ml/1 tsp sesame oil

2 spring onions (scallions), chopped

Bring the wine, water, soy sauce, sugar, salt and pepper to the boil and boil until reduced by half. Mix the cornflour to a paste with the water, stir it into the pan and simmer, stirring, for 2 minutes. Season the fish with salt and sprinkle with sesame oil. Add to the pan and simmer very gently for about 8 minutes until cooked. Serve sprinkled with spring onions.

Quick-Fried Fish

Serves 4

450 g/1 lb cod fillets, cut into strips

salt

soy sauce

oil for deep-frying

Sprinkle the fish with salt and soy sauce and leave to stand for 10 minutes. Heat the oil and deep-fry the fish for a few minutes until lightly golden. Drain on kitchen paper and sprinkle generously with soy sauce before serving.

Sesame Seed Fish

Serves 4

450 g/1 lb fish fillets, cut into strips

1 onion, chopped

2 slices ginger root, minced

120 ml/4 fl oz/¬Ω cup rice wine or dry sherry

10 ml/2 tsp brown sugar

2.5 ml/¬Ω tsp salt

1 egg, lightly beaten

15 ml/1 tbsp cornflour (cornstarch)

45 ml/3 tbsp plain (all-purpose) flour

60 ml/6 tbsp sesame seeds

oil for deep-frying

Place the fish in a bowl. Mix together the onion, ginger, wine or sherry, sugar and salt, add to the fish and leave to marinate for 30 minutes, turning occasionally. Beat the egg, cornflour and flour to make a batter. Dip the fish in the batter then press into the sesame seeds. Heat the oil and deep-fry the fish strips for about 1 minute until golden and crispy.

Steamed Fish Balls

Serves 4

450 g/1 lb minced (ground) cod

1 egg, lightly beaten

1 slice ginger root, minced

2.5 ml/¬Ω tsp salt

pinch of freshly ground pepper

15 ml/1 tbsp cornflour (cornstarch) 15 ml/1 tbsp rice wine or dry sherry

Mix all the ingredients together well and shape into walnut-sized balls. Dust with a little flour if necessary. Arrange in a shallow ovenproof dish.

Stand the dish on a rack in a steamer, cover and steam over gently simmering water for about 10 minutes until cooked.

Marinated Sweet and Sour Fish

Serves 4

450 g/1 lb fish fillets, cut into chunks

1 onion, chopped

3 slices ginger root, minced

5 ml/1 tsp soy sauce

salt and freshly ground pepper

30 ml/2 tbsp cornflour (cornstarch)

oil for deep-frying

sweet and sour sauce

Place the fish in a bowl. Mix together the onion, ginger, soy sauce, salt and pepper, add to the fish, cover and leave to stand for 1 hour, turning occasionally. Remove the fish from the marinade and dust with cornflour. Heat the oil and deep-fry the fish until crisp and golden brown. Drain on kitchen paper and arrange on a warmed serving plate. Meanwhile, prepare the sauce and pour over the fish to serve.

Fish with Vinegar Sauce

Serves 4

450 g/1 lb fish fillets, cut into strips

salt and freshly ground pepper

1 egg white, lightly beaten

45 ml/3 tbsp cornflour (cornstarch)

15 ml/1 tbsp rice wine or dry sherry

oil for deep-frying

250 ml/8 fl oz/1 cup fish stock

15 ml/1 tbsp brown sugar

15 ml/1 tbsp wine vinegar

2 slices root ginger, minced

2 spring onions (scallions), minced

Season the fish with a little salt and pepper. Beat the egg white with 30 ml/2 tbsp of cornflour and the wine or sherry. Toss the fish in the batter until coated. Heat the oil and deep-fry the fish for a few minutes until golden brown. Drain on kitchen paper.

Meanwhile, bring the stock, sugar and wine vinegar to the boil. Add the ginger and spring onion and simmer for 3 minutes. Blend the remaining cornflour to a paste with a little water, stir it into the pan and simmer, stirring, until the sauce clears and thickens. Pour over the fish to serve.

Deep-Fried Eel

Serves 4

450 g/1 lb eel

250 ml/8 fl oz/1 cup groundnut (peanut) oil

30 ml/2 tbsp dark soy sauce

30 ml/2 tbsp rice wine or dry sherry

15 ml/1 tbsp brown sugar

dash of sesame oil

Skin the eel and cut it into chunks. Heat the oil and fry the eel until golden. Remove from the pan and drain. Pour off all but 30 ml/2 tbsp of oil. Reheat the oil and add the soy sauce, wine or sherry and sugar. Heat through then add the eel and stir-fry until the eel is well coated and almost all the liquid has evaporated. Sprinkle with sesame oil and serve.

Dry-Cooked Eel

Serves 4

5 dried Chinese mushrooms

3 spring onions (scallions)

30 ml/2 tbsp groundnut (peanut) oil

20 cloves garlic

6 slices ginger root

10 water chestnuts

900 g/2 lb eels

30 ml/2 tbsp soy sauce

15 ml/1 tbsp brown sugar

15 ml/1 tbsp rice wine or dry sherry

450 ml/¬œ pt/2 cups water

15 ml/1 tbsp cornflour (cornstarch)

45 ml/3 tbsp water

5 ml/1 tsp sesame oil

Soak the mushrooms in warm water for 30 minutes then drain and discard the stalks. Cut 1 spring onion into chunks and chop the other. Heat the oil and fry the mushrooms, spring onion chunks, garlic, ginger and chestnuts for 30 seconds. Add the eels and stir-fry for 1 minute. Add the soy sauce, sugar, wine or

sherry and water, bring to the boil, cover and simmer gently for
1¬Ω hours, adding a little water during cooking if necessary.
Blend the cornflour and water to a paste, stir into the pan and
simmer, stirring, until the sauce thickens. Serve sprinkled with
sesame oil and the chopped spring onions.

Eel with Celery

Serves 4

350 g/12 oz eel

6 stalks celery

30 ml/2 tbsp groundnut (peanut) oil

2 spring onions (scallions), chopped

1 slice ginger root, minced

30 ml/2 tbsp water

5 ml/1 tsp sugar

5 ml/1 tsp rice wine or dry sherry

5 ml/1 tsp soy sauce

freshly ground pepper

30 ml/2 tbsp chopped fresh parsley

Skin and cut the eel into strips. Cut the celery into strips. Heat the oil and fry the spring onions and ginger for 30 seconds. Add the eel and stir-fry for 30 seconds. Add the celery and stir-fry for 30 seconds. Add half the water, the sugar, wine or sherry, soy sauce and pepper. Bring to the boil and simmer for a few minutes until the celery is just tender but still crisp and the liquid has reduced. Serve sprinkled with parsley.

Haddock-Stuffed Peppers

Serves 4

225 g/8 oz haddock fillets, minced (ground)

100 g/4 oz peeled prawns, minced (ground)

1 spring onion (scallion), chopped

2.5 ml/¬Ω tsp salt

pepper

4 green peppers

45 ml/3 tbsp groundnut (peanut) oil

120 ml/4 fl oz/¬Ω cup chicken stock

10 ml/2 tsp cornflour (cornstarch)

5 ml/1 tsp soy sauce

Mix together the haddock, prawns, spring onion, salt and pepper. Cut off the stem of the peppers and lift out the centre. Stuff the peppers with the seafood mixture. Heat the oil and add the peppers and stock. Bring to the boil, cover and simmer for 15 minutes. Transfer the peppers to a warmed serving plate. Mix the cornflour, soy sauce and a little water and stir it into the pan. Bring to the boil and simmer, stirring, until the sauce clears and thickens.

Haddock in Black Bean Sauce

Serves 4

15 ml/1 tbsp groundnut (peanut) oil

2 cloves garlic, crushed

1 slice ginger root, minced

15 ml/1 tbsp black bean sauce

2 onions, cut into wedges

1 stick celery, sliced

450 g/1 lb haddock fillets

15 ml/1 tbsp soy sauce

15 ml/1 tbsp rice wine or dry sherry

250 ml/8 fl oz/1 cup chicken stock

Heat the oil and fry the garlic, ginger and black bean sauce until lightly browned. Add the onions and celery and stir-fry for 2 minutes. Add the haddock and fry for about 4 minutes each side or until the fish is cooked. Add the soy sauce, wine or sherry and chicken stock, bring to the boil, cover and simmer for 3 minutes.

Fish in Brown Sauce

Serves 4

4 haddock or similar fish

45 ml/3 tbsp groundnut (peanut) oil

2 spring onions (scallions), chopped

2 slices ginger root, chopped

5 ml/1 tsp soy sauce

2.5 ml/¬Ω tsp wine vinegar

2.5 ml/¬Ω tsp rice wine or dry sherry

2.5 ml/¬Ω tsp sugar

freshly ground pepper

2.5 ml/¬Ω tsp sesame oil

Trim the fish and cut into large chunks. Heat the oil and fry the spring onions and ginger for 30 seconds. Add the fish and fry until lightly browned on both sides. Add the soy sauce, wine vinegar, wine or sherry, sugar and pepper and simmer for 5 minutes until the sauce is thick. Serve sprinkled with sesame oil.

Five-Spice Fish

Serves 4

450 g/1 lb haddock fillets

5 ml/1 tsp five-spice powder

5 ml/1 tsp salt

30 ml/2 tbsp groundnut (peanut) oil

2 cloves garlic, crushed

2 slices ginger root, minced

30 ml/2 tbsp rice wine or dry sherry

15 ml/1 tbsp soy sauce

10 ml/2 tsp sesame oil

Rub the haddock fillets with the five-spice powder and salt. Heat the oil and fry the fish until lightly browned on both sides then remove it from the pan. Add the garlic, ginger, wine or sherry, soy sauce and sesame oil and fry for 1 minute. Return the fish to the pan and simmer gently until the fish is tender.

Serves 4

450 g/1 lb haddock fillets

5 ml/1 tsp salt

30 ml/2 tbsp cornflour (cornstarch)

60 ml/4 tbsp groundnut (peanut) oil

6 cloves garlic

2 slices ginger root, crushed

45 ml/3 tbsp water

30 ml/2 tbsp soy sauce

15 ml/1 tbsp yellow bean sauce

15 ml/1 tbsp rice wine or dry sherry

15 ml/1 tbsp brown sugar

Sprinkle the haddock with salt and dust with cornflour. Heat the oil and fry the fish until golden brown on both sides then remove it from the pan. Add the garlic and ginger and fry for 1 minute. Add the remaining ingredients, bring to the boil, cover and simmer for 5 minutes. Return the fish to the pan, cover and simmer until tender.

Hot-Spiced Fish

Serves 4

450 g/1 lb haddock fillets, diced

juice of 1 lemon

30 ml/2 tbsp soy sauce

30 ml/2 tbsp oyster sauce

15 ml/1 tbsp grated lemon rind

pinch of ground ginger

salt and pepper

2 egg whites

45 ml/3 tbsp cornflour (cornstarch)

6 dried Chinese mushrooms

oil for deep-frying

5 spring onions (scallions), cut into strips

1 stick celery, cut into strips

100 g/4 oz bamboo shoots, cut into strips

250 ml/8 fl oz/1 cup chicken stock

5 ml/1 tsp five-spice powder

Put the fish in a bowl and sprinkle with lemon juice. Mix together the soy sauce, oyster sauce, lemon rind, ginger, salt, pepper, egg whites and all but 5 ml/1 tsp of the cornflour. Leave to marinate for 2 hours, stirring occasionally. Soak the mushrooms in warm water for 30 minutes then drain. Discard the stalks and slice the caps. Heat the oil and fry the fish for a few minutes until golden. Remove from the pan. Add the vegetables and fry until tender but still crisp. Pour off the oil. Mix the chicken stock with the remaining cornflour, add it to the vegetables and bring to the boil. Return the fish to the pan, season with five-spice powder and heat through before serving.

Ginger Haddock with Pak Soi

Serves 4

450 g/1 lb haddock fillet

salt and pepper

225 g/8 oz pak soi

30 ml/2 tbsp groundnut (peanut) oil

1 slice ginger root, chopped

1 onion, chopped

2 dried red chilli peppers

5 ml/1 tsp honey

10 ml/2 tsp tomato ketchup (catsup)

10 ml/2 tsp malt vinegar

30 ml/2 tbsp dry white wine

10 ml/2 tsp soy sauce

10 ml/2 tsp fish sauce

10 ml/2 tsp oyster sauce

5 ml/1 tsp shrimp paste

Skin the haddock then cut into 2 cm/ ¬æ in pieces. Sprinkle with salt and pepper. Cut the cabbage into small pieces. Heat the oil and fry the ginger and onion for 1 minute. Add the cabbage and chilli peppers and fry for 30 seconds. Add the honey, tomato ketchup, vinegar and wine. Add the haddock and simmer for 2 minutes. Stir in the soy, fish and oyster sauces and the shrimp paste and simmer gently until the haddock is cooked.

Haddock Plaits

Serves 4

450 g/1 lb haddock fillets, skinned

salt

5 ml/1 tsp five-spice powder

juice of 2 lemons

5 ml/1 tsp aniseed, ground

5 ml/1 tsp freshly ground pepper

30 ml/2 tbsp soy sauce

30 ml/2 tbsp oyster sauce

15 ml/1 tbsp honey

60 ml/4 tbsp chopped chives

8,Äì10 spinach leaves

45 ml/3 tbsp wine vinegar

Cut the fish into long thin strips and shape into plaits, sprinkle with salt, five-spice powder and lemon juice and transfer to a bowl. Mix together the aniseed, pepper, soy sauce, oyster sauce, honey and chives, pour over the fish and leave to marinate for at least 30 minutes. Line the steam basket with the spinach leaves, place the plaits on top, cover and steam over gently boiling water with the vinegar for about 25 minutes.

Steamed Fish Roulades

Serves 4

450 g/1 lb haddock fillets, skinned and diced

juice of 1 lemon

30 ml/2 tbsp soy sauce

30 ml/2 tbsp oyster sauce

30 ml/2 tbsp plum sauce

5 ml/1 tsp rice wine or dry sherry

salt and pepper

6 dried Chinese mushrooms

100 g/4 oz bean sprouts

100 g/4 oz green peas

50 g/2 oz/¬Ω cup walnuts, chopped

1 egg, beaten

30 ml/2 tbsp cornflour (cornstarch)

225 g/8 oz Chinese cabbage, blanched

Put the fish in a bowl. Mix together the lemon juice, soy, oyster and plum sauces, wine or sherry and salt and pepper. Pour over the fish and leave to marinate for 30 minutes. Add the vegetables, nuts, egg and cornflour and mix together well. Lay 3 Chinese leaves on top of each other, spoon on some of the fish mixture and roll up. Continue until all the ingredients have been used up. Place the rolls in a steam basket, cover and cook over gently simmering water for 30 minutes.

Halibut with Tomato Sauce

Serves 4

450 g/1 lb halibut fillets

salt

15 ml/1 tbsp black bean sauce

1 clove garlic, crushed

2 spring onions (scallions), chopped

2 slices ginger root, minced

15 ml/1 tbsp rice wine or dry sherry

15 ml/1 tbsp soy sauce

200 g/7 oz canned tomatoes, drained

30 ml/2 tbsp groundnut (peanut) oil

Sprinkle the halibut generously with salt and leave to stand for 1 hour. Rinse off the salt and pat dry. Place the fish in an ovenproof bowl and sprinkle with the black bean sauce, garlic, spring onions, ginger, wine or sherry, soy sauce and tomatoes. Place the bowl on a rack in a steamer, cover and steam for 20 minutes over boiling water until the fish is cooked. Heat the oil until almost smoking and sprinkle over the fish before serving.

Monkfish with Broccoli

Serves 4

450 g/1 lb monkfish tail, cubed

salt and pepper

45 ml/3 tbsp groundnut (peanut) oil

50 g/2 oz mushrooms, sliced

1 small carrot, cut into strips

1 clove garlic, crushed

2 slices ginger root, minced

45 ml/3 tbsp water

275 g/10 oz broccoli florets

5 ml/1 tsp sugar

5 ml/1 tsp cornflour (cornstarch)

45 ml/3 tbsp water

Season the monkfish well with salt and pepper. Heat 30 ml/2 tbsp of oil and fry the monkfish, mushrooms, carrot, garlic and ginger until lightly browned. Add the water and continue to simmer, uncovered, over a low heat. Meanwhile, blanch the broccoli in boiling water until just tender then drain well. Heat the remaining oil and stir-fry the broccoli and sugar with a pinch of salt until the broccoli is well coated in the oil. Arrange round a warmed serving plate. Mix the cornflour and water to a paste, stir into the fish and simmer, stirring, until the sauce thickens. Pour over the broccoli and serve at once.

Mullet with Thick Soy Sauce

Serves 4

1 red mullet

oil for deep-frying

30 ml/2 tbsp groundnut (peanut) oil

2 spring onions (scallions), sliced

2 slices ginger root, shredded

1 red chilli pepper, shredded

250 ml/8 fl oz/1 cup fish stock

15 ml/1 tbsp thick soy sauce

15 ml/1 tbsp freshly ground white

pepper

15 ml/1 tbsp rice wine or dry sherry

Trim the fish and score it diagonally on each side. Heat the oil and deep-fry the fish until half cooked. Remove from the oil and drain well. Heat the oil and fry the spring onions, ginger and chilli pepper for 1 minute. Add the remaining ingredients, stir together well and bring to the boil. Add the fish and simmer gently, uncovered, until the fish is cooked and the liquid has almost evaporated.

West Lake Fish

Serves 4

1 mullet

30 ml/2 tbsp groundnut (peanut) oil

4 spring onions (scallions), shredded

1 red chilli pepper, chopped

4 slices ginger root, shredded

45 ml/3 tbsp brown sugar

30 ml/2 tbsp red wine vinegar

30 ml/2 tbsp water

30 ml/2 tbsp soy sauce

freshly ground pepper

Clean and trim the fish and make 2 or 3 diagonal cuts on each side. Heat the oil and stir-fry half the spring onions, the chilli pepper and ginger for 30 seconds. Add the fish and fry until lightly browned on both sides. Add the sugar, wine vinegar, water, soy sauce and pepper, bring to the boil, cover and simmer for about 20 minutes until the fish is cooked and the sauce has reduced. Serve garnished with the remaining spring onions.

Fried Plaice

Serves 4

4 plaice fillets
salt and freshly ground pepper
30 ml/2 tbsp groundnut (peanut) oil
1 slice ginger root, minced
1 clove garlic, crushed
lettuce leaves

Season the plaice generously with salt and pepper. Heat the oil and fry the ginger and garlic for 20 seconds. Add the fish and fry until cooked through and golden brown. Drain well and serve on a bed of lettuce.

Steamed Plaice with Chinese Mushrooms

Serves 4

4 dried Chinese mushrooms

450 g/1 lb plaice fillets, cubed

1 clove garlic, crushed

1 slice ginger root, minced

15 ml/1 tbsp soy sauce

15 ml/1 tbsp rice wine or dry sherry

5 ml/1 tsp brown sugar

350 g/12 oz cooked long-grain rice

Soak the mushrooms in warm water for 30 minutes then drain. Discard the stems and chop the caps. Mix with the plaice, garlic, ginger, soy sauce, wine or sherry and sugar, cover and leave to marinate for 1 hour. Place the rice in a steamer and arrange the fish on top. Steam for about 30 minutes until the fish is cooked.

Plaice with Garlic

Serves 4

350 g/12 oz plaice fillets

salt

45 ml/3 tbsp cornflour (cornstarch)

1 egg, beaten

60 ml/4 tbsp groundnut (peanut) oil

3 cloves garlic, chopped

4 spring onions (scallions), chopped

15 ml/1 tbsp rice wine or dry sherry

5 ml/1 tsp sesame oil

Skin the plaice and cut it into strips. Sprinkle with salt and leave to stand for 20 minutes. Dust the fish with cornflour then dip in the egg. Heat the oil and fry the fish strips for about 4 minutes until golden brown. Remove from the pan and drain on kitchen paper. Pour off all but 5 ml/1 tsp of oil from the pan and add the remaining ingredients. Bring to the boil, stirring, then simmer for 3 minutes. Pour over the fish and serve immediately.

Plaice with Pineapple Sauce

Serves 4

450 g/1 lb plaice fillets

5 ml/1 tsp salt

30 ml/2 tbsp soy sauce

200 g/7 oz canned pineapple chunks

2 eggs, beaten

100 g/4 oz/¬Ω cup cornflour (cornstarch)

oil for deep-frying

30 ml/2 tbsp water

5 ml/1 tsp sesame oil

Cut the plaice into strips and place in a bowl. Sprinkle with salt, soy sauce and 30 ml/2 tbsp of the pineapple juice and leave to stand for 10 minutes. Beat the eggs with 45 ml/3 tbsp of cornflour to a batter and dip the fish in the batter. Heat the oil and deep-fry the fish until golden brown. Drain on kitchen pepper. Put the remaining pineapple juice in a small saucepan. Blend 30 ml/2 tbsp of cornflour with the water and stir it into the pan. Bring to the boil and simmer, stirring, until thickened. Add half the pineapple pieces and heat through. Just before serving, stir in the sesame oil. Arrange the cooked fish on a warmed serving plate and garnish with the reserved pineapple. Pour over the hot sauce and serve at once.

Salmon with Tofu

Serves 4

120 ml/4 fl oz/¬Ω cup groundnut (peanut) oil

450 g/1 lb tofu, cubed

2.5 ml/¬Ω tsp sesame oil

100 g/4 oz salmon fillet, chopped

dash of chilli sauce

250 ml/8 fl oz/1 cup fish stock

15 ml/1 tbsp cornflour (cornstarch)

45 ml/3 tbsp water

2 spring onions (scallions), chopped

Heat the oil and fry the tofu until lightly browned. Remove from the pan. Reheat the oil and sesame oil and fry the salmon and chilli sauce for 1 minute. Add the stock, bring to the boil, then return the tofu to the pan. Simmer gently, uncovered, until the ingredients are cooked through and the liquid has reduced. Blend the cornflour and water to a paste. Stir in a little at a time and simmer, stirring, until the mixture thickens. You may not need all the cornflour paste if you have allowed the liquid to reduce. Transfer to a warmed serving plate and sprinkle with the spring onions.

Deep-Fried Marinated Fish

Serves 4

450 g/1 lb sprats or other small fish, cleaned

3 slices ginger root, minced

120 ml/4 fl oz/¬Ω cup soy sauce

15 ml/1 tbsp rice wine or dry sherry

1 clove star anise

oil for deep-frying

15 ml/1 tbsp sesame oil

Place the fish in a bowl. Mix together the ginger, soy sauce, wine or sherry and anise, pour over the fish and leave to stand for 1 hour, turning occasionally. Drain the fish, discarding the marinade. Heat the oil and fry the fish in batches until crispy and golden brown. Drain on kitchen paper and serve sprinkled with sesame oil.

Trout with Carrots

Serves 4

15 ml/1 tbsp groundnut (peanut) oil

1 clove garlic, crushed

1 slice ginger root, minced

4 trout

2 carrots, cut into strips

25 g/1 oz bamboo shoots, cut into strips

25 g/1 oz water chestnuts, cut into strips

15 ml/1 tbsp soy sauce

15 ml/1 tbsp rice wine or dry sherry

Heat the oil and fry the garlic and ginger until lightly browned. Add the fish, cover and fry until the fish turns opaque. Add the carrots, bamboo shoots, chestnuts, soy sauce and wine or sherry, stir carefully, cover and simmer for about 5 minutes.

Deep-Fried Trout

Serves 4

4 trout, cleaned and scaled

2 eggs, beaten

50 g/2 oz/¬Ω cup plain (all-purpose) flour

oil for deep-frying

1 lemon, cut into wedges

Slash the fish diagonally a few times on each side. Dip in the beaten eggs then toss in the flour to coat completely. Shake off any excess. Heat the oil and deep-fry the fish for about 10 to 15 minutes until cooked. Drain on kitchen paper and serve with lemon.

Trout with Lemon Sauce

Serves 4

450 ml/¬œ pt/2 cups chicken stock

5 cm/2 in square piece lemon rind

150 ml/¬° pt/generous ¬Ω cup lemon juice

90 ml/6 tbsp brown sugar

2 slices ginger root, cut into strips

30 ml/2 tbsp cornflour (cornstarch)

4 trout

375 g/12 oz/3 cups plain (all-purpose) flour

175 ml/6 fl oz/¬œ cup water

oil for deep-frying

2 egg whites

8 spring onions (scallions), thinly sliced

To make the sauce, mix together the stock, lemon rind and juice, sugar and for 5 minutes. Remove from the heat, strain and return to the pan. Mix the cornflour with a little water then stir it into the pan. Simmer for 5 minutes, stirring frequently. Remove from the heat and keep the sauce warm.

Lightly coat the fish on both sides with a little of the flour. Beat the remaining flour with the water and 10 ml/2 tsp of oil until smooth. Beat the egg whites until stiff but not dry and fold them into the batter. Heat the remaining oil. Dip the fish in the batter to coat it completely. Cook the fish for about 10 minutes, turning once, until cooked through and golden. Drain on kitchen paper. Arrange the fish on a warmed serving plate. Stir the spring onions into the warm sauce, pour over the fish and serve immediately.

Chinese Tuna

Serves 4

30 ml/2 tbsp groundnut (peanut) oil
1 onion, chopped
200 g/7 oz canned tuna, drained and flaked
2 stalks celery, chopped
100 g/4 oz mushrooms, chopped
1 green pepper, chopped
250 ml/8 fl oz/1 cup stock
30 ml/2 tbsp soy sauce
100 g/4 oz fine egg noodles
salt
15 ml/1 tbsp cornflour (cornstarch)
45 ml/3 tbsp water

Heat the oil and fry the onion until softened. Add the tuna and stir until well coated with oil. Add the celery, mushrooms and pepper and stir-fry for 2 minutes. Add the stock and soy sauce, bring to the boil, cover and simmer for 15 minutes. Meanwhile, cook the noodles in boiling salt water for about 5 minutes until just tender then drain well and arrange on a warmed serving plate. Mix the cornflour and water, stir the mixture into the tuna sauce and simmer, stirring, until the sauce clears and thickens.

Marinated Fish Steaks

Serves 4

4 whiting or haddock steaks
2 cloves garlic, crushed
2 slices ginger root, crushed
3 spring onions (scallions), chopped
15 ml/1 tbsp rice wine or dry sherry
15 ml/1 tbsp wine vinegar
salt and freshly ground pepper
45 ml/3 tbsp groundnut (peanut) oil

Place the fish in a bowl. Mix the garlic, ginger, spring onions, wine or sherry, wine vinegar, salt and pepper, pour over the fish, cover and leave to marinate for several hours. Remove the fish from the marinade. Heat the oil and fry the fish until browned on both sides then remove from the pan. Add the marinade to the pan, bring to the boil then return the fish to the pan and simmer gently until cooked through.

Prawns with Almonds

Serves 4

100 g/4 oz almonds

225 g/8 oz large unpeeled prawns

2 slices ginger root, minced

15 ml/1 tbsp cornflour (cornstarch)

2.5 ml/¬Ω tsp salt

30 ml/2 tbsp groundnut (peanut) oil

2 cloves garlic

2 stalks celery, chopped

5 ml/1 tsp soy sauce

5 ml/1 tsp rice wine or dry sherry

30 ml/2 tbsp water

Toast the almonds in a dry pan until lightly browned then put to one side. Peel the prawns, leaving on the tails, and cut in half lengthways to the tail. Mix with the ginger, cornflour and salt. Heat the oil and fry the garlic until lightly browned then discard the garlic. Add the celery, soy sauce, wine or sherry and water to the pan and bring to the boil. Add the prawns and stir-fry until heated through. Serve sprinkled with toasted almonds.

Anise Prawns

Serves 4

45 ml/3 tbsp groundnut (peanut) oil
15 ml/1 tbsp soy sauce
5 ml/1 tsp sugar
120 ml/4 fl oz/¬Ω cup fish stock
pinch of ground anise
450 g/1 lb peeled prawns

Heat the oil, add the soy sauce, sugar, stock and anise and bring to the boil. Add the prawns and simmer for a few minutes until heated through and flavoured.

Prawns with Asparagus

Serves 4

450 g/1 lb asparagus, cut into chunks

45 ml/3 tbsp groundnut (peanut) oil

2 slices ginger root, minced

15 ml/1 tbsp soy sauce

15 ml/1 tbsp rice wine or dry sherry

5 ml/1 tsp sugar

2.5 ml/¬Ω tsp salt

225 g/8 oz peeled prawns

Blanch the asparagus in boiling water for 2 minutes then drain well. Heat the oil and fry the ginger for a few seconds. Add the asparagus and stir until well coated with oil. Add the soy sauce, wine or sherry, sugar and salt and heat through. Add the prawns and stir over a low heat until the asparagus is tender.

Prawns with Bacon

Serves 4

450 g/1 lb large unpeeled prawns

100 g/4 oz bacon

1 egg, lightly beaten

2.5 ml/¬Ω tsp salt

15 ml/1 tbsp soy sauce

50 g/2 oz/¬Ω cup cornflour (cornstarch)

oil for deep-frying

Peel the prawns, leaving the tails intact. Cut in half lengthways to the tail. Cut the bacon into small squares. Press a piece of bacon in the centre of each prawn and press the two halves together. Beat the egg with the salt and soy sauce. Dip the prawns in the egg then dust with cornflour. Heat the oil and deep-fry the prawns until crispy and golden.

Prawn Balls

Serves 4

3 dried Chinese mushrooms

450 g/1 lb prawns, finely minced

6 water chestnuts, finely minced

1 spring onion (scallion), finely minced

1 slice ginger root, finely minced

salt and freshly ground pepper

2 eggs, beaten

15 ml/1 tbsp cornflour (cornstarch)

50 g/2 oz/¬Ω cup plain (all-purpose) flour

groundnut (peanut) oil for deep-frying

Soak the mushrooms in warm water for 30 minutes then drain. Discard the stems and finely chop the caps. Mix with the prawns, water chestnuts, spring onion and ginger and season with salt and pepper. Mix in 1 egg and 5 ml/1 tsp cornflour roll into balls about the size of a heaped teaspoon.

Beat together the remaining egg, cornflour and flour and add enough water to make a thick, smooth batter. Roll the balls in the batter. Heat the oil and deep-fry for a few minutes until light golden brown.

Barbecued Prawns

Serves 4

450 g/1 lb large peeled prawns

100 g/4 oz bacon

225 g/8 oz chicken livers, sliced

1 clove garlic, crushed

2 slices ginger root, minced

30 ml/2 tbsp sugar

120 ml/4 fl oz/¬Ω cup soy sauce

salt and freshly ground pepper

Cut the prawns lengthways down the back without cutting right through and flatten them slightly. Cut the bacon into chunks and place in a bowl with the prawns and chicken livers. Mix together the remaining ingredients, pour over the prawns and leave to stand for 30 minutes. Thread the prawns, bacon and livers oh to skewers and grill or barbecue for about 5 minutes, turning frequently, until cooked through, basting occasionally with the marinade.

Prawns with Bamboo Shoots

Serves 4

60 ml/4 tbsp groundnut (peanut) oil

1 clove garlic, minced

1 slice ginger root, minced

450 g/1 lb peeled prawns

30 ml/2 tbsp rice wine or dry sherry

225 g/8 oz bamboo shoots

30 ml/2 tbsp soy sauce

15 ml/1 tbsp cornflour (cornstarch)

45 ml/3 tbsp water

Heat the oil and fry the garlic and ginger until lightly browned. Add the prawns and stir-fry for 1 minute. Add the wine or sherry and stir together well. Add the bamboo shoots and stir-fry for 5 minutes. Add the remaining ingredients and stir-fry for 2 minutes.

Prawns with Bean Sprouts

Serves 4

4 dried Chinese mushrooms

30 ml/2 tbsp groundnut (peanut) oil

1 clove garlic, crushed

225 g/8 oz peeled prawns

15 ml/1 tbsp rice wine or dry sherry

450 g/1 lb bean sprouts

120 ml/4 fl oz/¬Ω cup chicken stock

15 ml/1 tbsp soy sauce

15 ml/1 tbsp cornflour (cornstarch)

salt and freshly ground pepper

2 spring onion (scallions), chopped

Soak the mushrooms in warm water for 30 minutes then drain. Discard the stems and slice the caps. Heat the oil and fry the garlic until lightly browned. Add the prawns and stir-fry for 1 minute. Add the wine or sherry and fry for 1 minute. Stir in the mushrooms and bean sprouts. Mix together the stock, soy sauce and cornflour and stir it into the pan. Bring to the boil then simmer, stirring, until the sauce clears and thickens. Season to taste with salt and pepper. Serve sprinkled with spring onions.

Prawns with Black Bean Sauce

Serves 4

30 ml/2 tbsp groundnut (peanut) oil
5 ml/1 tsp salt
1 clove garlic, crushed
45 ml/3 tbsp black bean sauce
1 green pepper, chopped
1 onion, chopped
120 ml/4 fl oz/¬Ω cup fish stock
5 ml/1 tsp sugar
15 ml/1 tbsp soy sauce
225 g/8 oz peeled prawns
15 ml/1 tbsp cornflour (cornstarch)
45 ml/3 tbsp water

Heat the oil and stir-fry the salt, garlic and black bean sauce for 2 minutes. Add the pepper and onion and stir-fry for 2 minutes. Add the stock, sugar and soy sauce and bring to the boil. Add the prawns and simmer for 2 minutes. Mix the cornflour and water to a paste, add it to the pan and simmer, stirring, until the sauce clears and thickens.

Prawns with Celery

Serves 4

45 ml/3 tbsp groundnut (peanut) oil

3 slices ginger root, minced

450 g/1 lb peeled prawns

5 ml/1 tsp salt

15 ml/1 tbsp sherry

4 stalks celery, chopped

100 g/4 oz almonds, chopped

Heat half the oil and fry the ginger until lightly browned. Add the prawns, salt and sherry and stir-fry until well coated in oil then remove from the pan. Heat the remaining oil and stir-fry the celery and almonds for a few minutes until the celery is just tender but still crisp. Return the prawns to the pan, mix well and heat through before serving.

Stir-Fried Prawns with Chicken

Serves 4

30 ml/2 tbsp groundnut (peanut) oil

2 cloves garlic, crushed

225 g/8 oz cooked chicken, thinly sliced

100 g/4 oz bamboo shoots, sliced

100 g/4 oz mushrooms, sliced

75 ml/5 tbsp fish stock

225 g/8 oz peeled prawns

225 g/8 oz mangetout (snow peas)

15 ml/1 tbsp cornflour (cornstarch)

45 ml/3 tbsp water

Heat the oil and fry the garlic until lightly browned. Add the chicken, bamboo shoots and mushrooms and stir-fry until well coated in oil. Add the stock and bring to the boil. Add the prawns and mangetout, cover and simmer for 5 minutes. Mix the cornflour and water to a paste, stir into the pan and simmer, stirring, until the sauce clears and thickens. Serve at once.

Chilli Prawns

Serves 4

450 g/1 lb peeled prawns

1 egg white

10 ml/2 tsp cornflour (cornstarch)

5 ml/1 tsp salt

60 ml/4 tbsp groundnut (peanut) oil

25 g/1 oz dried red chilli peppers, trimmed

1 clove garlic, crushed

5 ml/1 tsp freshly ground pepper

15 ml/1 tbsp soy sauce

5 ml/1 tsp rice wine or dry sherry

2.5 ml/¬Ω tsp sugar

2.5 ml/¬Ω tsp wine vinegar

2.5 ml/¬Ω tsp sesame oil

Place the prawns in a bowl with the egg white, cornflour and salt and leave to marinate for 30 minutes. Heat the oil and fry the chilli peppers, garlic and pepper for 1 minute. Add the prawns and remaining ingredients and stir-fry for a few minutes until the prawns are heated through and the ingredients well mixed.

Prawn Chop Suey

Serves 4

60 ml/4 tbsp groundnut (peanut) oil

2 spring onions (scallions), chopped

2 cloves garlic, crushed

1 slice ginger root, chopped

225 g/8 oz peeled prawns

100 g/4 oz frozen peas

100 g/4 oz button mushrooms, halved

30 ml/2 tbsp soy sauce

15 ml/1 tbsp rice wine or dry sherry

5 ml/1 tsp sugar

5 ml/1 tsp salt

15 ml/1 tbsp cornflour (cornstarch)

Heat 45 ml/3 tbsp of oil and fry the spring onions, garlic and ginger until lightly browned. Add the prawns and stir-fry for 1 minute. Remove from the pan. Heat the remaining oil and stir-fry the peas and mushrooms for 3 minutes. Add the prawns, soy sauce, wine or sherry, sugar and salt and stir-fry for 2 minutes. Mix the cornflour with a little water, stir it into the pan and simmer, stirring, until the sauce clears and thickens.

Prawn Chow Mein

Serves 4

450 g/1 lb peeled prawns

15 ml/1 tbsp cornflour (cornstarch)

15 ml/1 tbsp soy sauce

15 ml/1 tbsp rice wine or dry sherry

4 dried Chinese mushrooms

30 ml/2 tbsp groundnut (peanut) oil

5 ml/1 tsp salt

1 slice ginger root, minced

100 g/4 oz Chinese cabbage, sliced

100 g/4 oz bamboo shoots, sliced

Soft-Fried Noodles

Mix the prawns with the cornflour, soy sauce and wine or sherry and leave to stand, stirring occasionally. Soak the mushrooms in warm water for 30 minutes then drain. Discard the stalks and slice the caps. Heat the oil and fry the salt and ginger for 1 minute. Add the cabbage and bamboo shoots and stir until coated with oil. Cover and simmer for 2 minutes. Stir in the prawns and marinade and stir-fry for 3 minutes. Stir in the drained noodles and heat through before serving.

Prawns with Courgettes and Lychees

Serves 4

12 king prawns

salt and pepper

10 ml/2 tsp soy sauce

10 ml/2 tsp cornflour (cornstarch)

15 ml/1 tbsp groundnut (peanut) oil

4 cloves garlic, crushed

2 red chilli peppers, chopped

225 g/8 oz courgettes (zucchini), diced

2 spring onions (scallions), chopped

12 lychees, stoned

120 ml/4 fl oz/¬Ω cup coconut cream

10 ml/2 tsp mild curry powder

5 ml/1 tsp fish sauce

Peel the prawns, leaving on the tails. Sprinkle with salt, pepper and soy sauce then coat with cornflour. Heat the oil and fry the garlic, chilli peppers and prawns for 1 minute. Add the courgettes, spring onions and lychees and stir-fry for 1 minute. Remove from the pan. Pour the coconut cream into the pan, bring to the boil and simmer for 2 minutes until thick. Stir in the curry powder and fish sauce and season with salt and pepper. Return the prawns and vegetables to the sauce to heat through before serving.

Prawns with Crab

Serves 4

45 ml/3 tbsp groundnut (peanut) oil

3 spring onions (scallions), chopped

1 sliced ginger root, minced

225 g/8 oz crab meat

15 ml/1 tbsp rice wine or dry sherry

30 ml/2 tbsp chicken or fish stock

15 ml/1 tbsp soy sauce

5 ml/1 tsp brown sugar

5 ml/1 tsp wine vinegar

freshly ground pepper

10 ml/2 tsp cornflour (cornstarch)

225 g/8 oz peeled prawns

Heat 30 ml/2 tbsp of oil and fry the spring onions and ginger until lightly browned. Add the crab meat and stir-fry for 2 minutes. Add the wine or sherry, stock, soy sauce, sugar and vinegar and season to taste with pepper. Stir-fry for 3 minutes. Mix the cornflour with a little water and stir it into the sauce. Simmer, stirring, until the sauce thickens. Meanwhile, heat the remaining oil in a separate pan and stir-fry the prawns for a few minutes until heated through. Arrange the crab mixture on a warmed serving plate and top with the prawns.

Prawns with Cucumber

Serves 4

225 g/8 oz peeled prawns

salt and freshly ground pepper

15 ml/1 tbsp cornflour (cornstarch)

1 cucumber

45 ml/3 tbsp groundnut (peanut) oil

2 cloves garlic, crushed

1 onion, finely chopped

15 ml/1 tbsp rice wine or dry sherry

2 slices ginger root, minced

Season the prawns with salt and pepper and toss with the cornflour. Peel and seed the cucumber and cut it into thick slices. Heat half the oil and fry the garlic and onion until lightly browned. Add the prawns and sherry and stir-fry for 2 minutes then remove the ingredients from the pan. Heat the remaining oil and fry the ginger for 1 minute. Add the cucumber and stir-fry for 2 minutes. Return the prawn mixture to the pan and stir-fry until well mixed and heated through.

Prawn Curry

Serves 4

45 ml/3 tbsp groundnut (peanut) oil

4 spring onions (scallions), sliced

30 ml/2 tbsp curry powder

2.5 ml/¬Ω tsp salt

120 ml/4 fl oz/¬Ω cup chicken stock

450 g/1 lb peeled prawns

Heat the oil and fry the spring onions for 30 seconds. Add the curry powder and salt and stir-fry for 1 minute. Add the stock, bring to the boil and simmer, stirring, for 2 minutes. Add the prawns and heat through gently.

Prawn and Mushroom Curry

Serves 4

5 ml/1 tsp soy sauce

5 ml/1 tsp rice wine or dry sherry

225 g/8 oz peeled prawns

30 ml/2 tbsp groundnut (peanut) oil

2 cloves garlic, crushed

1 slice ginger root, finely chopped

1 onion, cut into wedges

100 g/4 oz button mushrooms

100 g/4 oz fresh or frozen peas

15 ml/1 tbsp curry powder

15 ml/1 tbsp cornflour (cornstarch)

150 ml/¬° pt/generous ¬Ω cup chicken stock

Mix together the soy sauce, wine or sherry and prawns. Heat the oil with the garlic and ginger and fry until lightly browned. Add the onion, mushrooms and peas and stir-fry for 2 minutes. Add the curry powder and cornflour and stir-fry for 2 minutes. Gradually stir in the stock, bring to the boil, cover and simmer for 5 minutes, stirring occasionally. Add the prawns and marinade, cover and simmer for 2 minutes.

Deep-Fried Prawns

Serves 4

450 g/1 lb peeled prawns

30 ml/2 tbsp rice wine or dry sherry

5 ml/1 tsp salt

oil for deep-frying

soy sauce

Toss the prawns in the wine or sherry and sprinkle with salt. Leave to stand for 15 minutes then drain and pat dry. Heat the oil and deep-fry the prawns for a few seconds until crisp. Serve sprinkled with soy sauce.

Deep-Fried Battered Prawns

Serves 4

50 g/2 oz/¬Ω cup plain (all-purpose) flour

2.5 ml/¬Ω tsp salt

1 egg, lightly beaten

30 ml/2 tbsp water

450 g/1 lb peeled prawns

oil for deep-frying

Beat the flour, salt, egg and water to a batter, adding a little more water if necessary. Mix with the prawns until well coated. Heat the oil and deep-fry the prawns for a few minutes until crispy and golden.

Prawn Dumplings with Tomato Sauce

Serves 4

900 g/2 lb peeled prawns

450 g/1 lb minced (ground) cod

4 eggs, beaten

50 g/2 oz/¬Ω cup cornflour (cornstarch)

2 cloves garlic, crushed

30 ml/2 tbsp soy sauce

15 ml/1 tbsp sugar

15 ml/1 tbsp groundnut (peanut) oil

For the sauce:

30 ml/2 tbsp groundnut (peanut) oil

100 g/4 oz spring onions (scallions), chopped

100 g/4 oz mushrooms, chopped

100 g/4 oz ham, chopped

2 stalks celery, chopped

200 g/7 oz tomatoes, skinned and chopped

300 ml/¬Ω pt/1¬° cups water

salt and freshly ground pepper

15 ml/1 tbsp cornflour (cornstarch)

Finely chop the prawns and mix with the cod. Stir in the eggs, cornflour, garlic, soy sauce, sugar and oil. Bring a large saucepan of water to the boil and drop spoonfuls of the mixture into the saucepan. Return to the boil and simmer for a few minutes until the dumplings float to the surface. Drain well. To make the sauce, heat the oil and fry the spring onions until soft but not browned. Add the mushrooms and fry for 1 minute then add the ham, celery and tomatoes and fry for 1 minute. Add the water, bring to the boil and season with salt and pepper. Cover and simmer for 10 minutes, stirring occasionally. Mix the cornflour with a little water and stir it into the sauce. Simmer for a few minutes, stirring, until the sauce clears and thickens. Serve with the dumplings.

Prawn and Egg Cups

Serves 4

15 ml/1 tbsp sesame oil

8 peeled king prawns

1 red chilli pepper, chopped

2 spring onions (scallions), chopped

30 ml/2 tbsp chopped abalone (optional)

8 eggs

15 ml/1 tbsp soy sauce

salt and freshly ground pepper

few sprigs of flat-leaved parsley

Use the sesame oil to grease 8 ramekin dishes. Place one prawn in each dish with a little of the chilli pepper, spring onions and abalone, if using. Break an egg into each bowl and season with soy sauce, salt and pepper. Stand the ramekins on a baking sheet and bake in a preheated oven at 200°C/400°F/gas mark 6 for about 15 minutes until the eggs are set and slightly crisp around the outside. Lift them carefully on to a warmed serving plate and garnish with parsley.

Prawn Egg Rolls

Serves 4

225 g/8 oz bean sprouts

30 ml/2 tbsp groundnut (peanut) oil

4 stalks celery, chopped

100 g/4 oz mushrooms, chopped

225 g/8 oz peeled prawns, chopped

15 ml/1 tbsp rice wine or dry sherry

2.5 ml/¬Ω tsp cornflour (cornstarch)

2.5 ml/¬Ω tsp salt

2.5 ml/¬Ω tsp sugar

12 egg roll skins

1 egg, beaten

oil for deep-frying

Blanch the bean sprouts in boiling water for 2 minutes then drain. Heat the oil and stir-fry the celery for 1 minute. Add the mushrooms and stir-fry for 1 minute. Add the prawns, wine or sherry, cornflour, salt and sugar and stir-fry for 2 minutes. Leave to cool.

Place a little of the filling on the centre of each skin and brush the edges with beaten egg. Fold in the edges then roll the egg roll away from you, sealing the edges with egg. Heat the oil and deep-fry until golden brown.

Far Eastern Style Prawns

Serves 4

16,Äì20 peeled king prawns

juice of 1 lemon

120 ml/4 fl oz/¬Ω cup dry white wine

30 ml/2 tbsp soy sauce

30 ml/2 tbsp honey

15 ml/1 tbsp grated lemon rind

salt and pepper

45 ml/3 tbsp groundnut (peanut) oil

1 clove garlic, chopped

6 spring onions (scallions), cut into strips

2 carrots, cut into strips

5 ml/1 tsp five-spice powder

5 ml/1 tsp cornflour (cornstarch)

Mix the prawns with the lemon juice, wine, soy sauce, honey and lemon rind and season with salt and pepper. Cover and marinate for 1 hour. Heat the oil and fry the garlic until lightly browned. Add the vegetables and stir-fry until tender but still crisp. Drain the prawns, add them to the pan and stir-fry for 2 minutes. Strain the marinade and mix it with the five-spice powder and cornflour. Add to the wok, stir well and bring to the boil.

Prawn Foo Yung

Serves 4

6 eggs, beaten

45 ml/3 tbsp cornflour (cornstarch)

225 g/8 oz peeled prawns

100 g/4 oz mushrooms, sliced

5 ml/1 tsp salt

2 spring onions (scallions), chopped

45 ml/3 tbsp groundnut (peanut) oil

Beat the eggs then beat in the cornflour. Add all the remaining ingredients except the oil. Heat the oil and pour the mixture into the pan a little at a time to make pancakes about 7.5 cm/3 in across. Fry until the bottom is golden brown then turn and brown the other side.

Prawn Fries

Serves 4

12 large uncooked prawns

1 egg, beaten

30 ml/2 tbsp cornflour (cornstarch)

pinch of salt

pinch of pepper

3 slices bread

1 hard-boiled (hard-cooked) egg yolk, chopped

25 g/1 oz cooked ham, chopped

1 spring onion (scallion), chopped

oil for deep-frying

Remove the shells and back veins from the prawns, leaving the tails intact. Cut down the back of the prawns with a sharp knife and gently press them flat. Beat the egg, cornflour, salt and pepper. Toss the prawns in the mixture until completely coated. Remove the crusts from the bread and cut it into quarters. Place one prawn, cut side down, on each piece and press down. Brush a little egg mixture over each prawn then sprinkle with the egg yolk, ham and spring onion. Heat the oil and fry the prawn bread pieces in batches until golden. Drain on kitchen paper and serve hot.

Fried Prawns in Sauce

Serves 4

75 g/3 oz/heaped ¬° cup cornflour (cornstarch)

¬Ω egg, beaten

5 ml/1 tsp rice wine or dry sherry

salt

450 g/1 lb peeled prawns

45 ml/3 tbsp groundnut (peanut) oil

5 ml/1 tsp sesame oil

1 clove garlic, crushed

1 slice ginger root, minced

3 spring onions (scallions), sliced

15 ml/1 tbsp fish stock

5 ml/1 tsp wine vinegar

5 ml/1 tsp sugar

Mix together the cornflour, egg, wine or sherry and a pinch of salt to make a batter. Dip the prawns in the batter so that they are lightly coated. Heat the oil and fry the prawns until they are crisp outside. Remove them from the pan and drain off the oil. Heat the sesame oil in the pan, add the prawns, garlic, ginger and spring onions and stir-fry for 3 minutes. Stir in the stock, wine vinegar and sugar, stir well and heat through before serving.

Poached Prawns with Ham and Tofu

Serves 4

30 ml/2 tbsp groundnut (peanut) oil
225 g/8 oz tofu, cubed
600 ml/1 pt/2¬Ω cups chicken stock
100 g/4 oz smoked ham, cubed
225 g/8 oz peeled prawns

Heat the oil and fry the tofu until lightly browned. Remove from the pan and drain. Heat the stock, add the tofu and ham and simmer gently for about 10 minutes until the tofu is cooked. Add the prawns and simmer for a further 5 minutes until heated through. Serve in deep bowls.

Prawns in Lobster Sauce

Serves 4

45 ml/3 tbsp groundnut (peanut) oil

2 cloves garlic, crushed

5 ml/1 tsp minced black beans

100 g/4 oz minced (ground) pork

450 g/1 lb peeled prawns

15 ml/1 tbsp rice wine or dry sherry

300 ml/¬Ω pt/1¬° cups chicken stock

30 ml/2 tbsp cornflour (cornstarch)

2 eggs, beaten

15 ml/1 tbsp soy sauce

2.5 ml/¬Ω tsp salt

2.5 ml/¬Ω tsp sugar

2 spring onions (scallions), chopped

Heat the oil and fry the garlic and black beans until the garlic is
until lightly browned. Add the pork and fry until browned. Add
the prawns and stir-fry for 1 minute. Add the sherry, cover and
simmer for 1 minute. Add the stock and cornflour, bring to the
boil, stirring, cover and simmer for 5 minutes. Add the eggs,
stirring all the time so that they form into threads. Add the soy

sauce, salt, sugar and spring onions and simmer for a few minutes before serving.

Serves 4

50 g/2 oz/¬Ω cup plain (all-purpose)
flour

2.5 ml/¬Ω tsp salt

1 egg, lightly beaten

30 ml/2 tbsp water

450 g/1 lb peeled prawns

oil for deep-frying

30 ml/2 tbsp groundnut (peanut) oil

2 slices ginger root, minced

30 ml/2 tbsp wine vinegar

5 ml/1 tsp sugar

2.5 ml/¬Ω tsp salt

15 ml/1 tbsp soy sauce

200 g/7 oz canned lychees, drained

Beat together the flour, salt, egg and water to make a batter, adding a little more water if necessary. Mix with the prawns until they are well coated. Heat the oil and deep-fry the prawns for a few minutes until crispy and golden. Drain on kitchen paper and arrange on a warmed serving plate. Meanwhile, heat the oil and fry the ginger for 1 minute. Add the wine vinegar, sugar, salt and soy sauce. Add the lychees and stir until warm and coated with sauce. Pour over the prawns and serve at once.

Mandarin Fried Prawns

Serves 4

60 ml/4 tbsp groundnut (peanut) oil
1 clove garlic, crushed
1 slice ginger root, minced
450 g/1 lb peeled prawns
30 ml/2 tbsp rice wine or dry sherry 30 ml/2 tbsp soy sauce
15 ml/1 tbsp cornflour (cornstarch)
45 ml/3 tbsp water

Heat the oil and fry the garlic and ginger until lightly browned. Add the prawns and stir-fry for 1 minute. Add the wine or sherry and stir together well. Add the soy sauce, cornflour and water and stir-fry for 2 minutes.

Prawns with Mangetout

Serves 4

5 dried Chinese mushrooms

225 g/8 oz bean sprouts

60 ml/4 tbsp groundnut (peanut) oil

5 ml/1 tsp salt

2 stalks celery, chopped

4 spring onions (scallions), chopped

2 cloves garlic, crushed

2 slices ginger root, minced

60 ml/4 tbsp water

15 ml/1 tbsp soy sauce

15 ml/1 tbsp rice wine or dry sherry

225 g/8 oz mangetout (snow peas)

225 g/8 oz peeled prawns

15 ml/1 tbsp cornflour (cornstarch)

Soak the mushrooms in warm water for 30 minutes then drain. Discard the stalks and slice the caps. Blanch the bean sprouts in boiling water for 5 minutes then drain well. Heat half the oil and fry the salt, celery, spring onions and bean sprouts for 1 minute then remove them from the pan. Heat the remaining oil and fry the garlic and ginger until lightly browned. Add half the water, the soy sauce, wine or sherry, mangetout and prawns, bring to the boil and simmer for 3 minutes. Mix the cornflour and remaining water to a paste, stir into the pan and simmer, stirring, until the sauce, thickens. Return the vegetables to the pan, simmer until heated through. Serve at once.

Prawns with Chinese Mushrooms

Serves 4

8 dried Chinese mushrooms

45 ml/3 tbsp groundnut (peanut) oil

3 slices ginger root, minced

450 g/1 lb peeled prawns

15 ml/1 tbsp soy sauce

5 ml/1 tsp salt

60 ml/4 tbsp fish stock

Soak the mushrooms in warm water for 30 minutes then drain. Discard the stalks and slice the caps. Heat half the oil and fry the ginger until lightly browned. Add the prawns, soy sauce and salt and stir-fry until coated in oil then remove from the pan. Heat the remaining oil and stir-fry the mushrooms until coated with oil.

Add the stock, bring to the boil, cover and simmer for 3 minutes. Return the prawns to the pan and stir until heated through.

Prawn and Pea Stir-Fry

Serves 4

450 g/1 lb peeled prawns

5 ml/1 tsp sesame oil

5 ml/1 tsp salt

30 ml/2 tbsp groundnut (peanut) oil

1 clove garlic, crushed

1 slice ginger root, minced

225 g/8 oz blanched or frozen peas, thawed

4 spring onions (scallions), chopped

30 ml/2 tbsp water

salt and pepper

Mix the prawns with the sesame oil and salt. Heat the oil and stir-fry the garlic and ginger for 1 minute. Add the prawns and stir-fry for 2 minutes. Add the peas and stir-fry for 1 minute. Add the spring onions and water and season with salt and pepper and a little more sesame oil, if liked. Heat through, stirring carefully, before serving.

Prawns with Mango Chutney

Serves 4

12 king prawns
salt and pepper
juice of 1 lemon
30 ml/2 tbsp cornflour (cornstarch)
1 mango
5 ml/1 tsp mustard powder
5 ml/1 tsp honey
30 ml/2 tbsp coconut cream
30 ml/2 tbsp mild curry powder
120 ml/4 fl oz/¬Ω cup chicken stock
45 ml/3 tbsp groundnut (peanut) oil
2 cloves garlic, chopped
2 spring onions (scallions), chopped
1 fennel bulb, chopped
100 g/4 oz mango chutney

Peel the prawns, leaving the tails intact. Sprinkle with salt, pepper and lemon juice then coat with half the cornflour. Peel the mango, cut the flesh away from the stone then dice the flesh. Mix the mustard, honey, coconut cream, curry powder, the remaining cornflour and the stock. Heat half the oil and fry the garlic, spring onions and fennel for 2 minutes. Add the stock mixture, bring to the boil and simmer for 1 minute. Add the mango cubes and chutney and heat through gently then transfer to a warmed serving plate. Heat the remaining oil and stir-fry the prawns for 2 minutes. Arrange them on the vegetables and serve at once.

Fried Prawn Balls with Onion Sauce

Serves 4

3 eggs, lightly beaten

45 ml/3 tbsp plain (all-purpose) flour

salt and freshly ground pepper

450 g/1 lb peeled prawns

oil for deep-frying

15 ml/1 tbsp groundnut (peanut) oil

2 onions, chopped

15 ml/1 tbsp cornflour (cornstarch)

30 ml/2 tbsp soy sauce

175 ml/6 fl oz/¬œ cup water

Mix the eggs, flour, salt and pepper. Toss the prawns in the batter. Heat the oil and deep-fry the prawns until golden brown. Meanwhile, heat the oil and fry the onions for 1 minute. Blend the remaining ingredients to a paste, stir into the onions and cook, stirring, until the sauce thickens. Drain the prawns and arrange on a warmed serving plate. Pour over the sauce and serve at once.

Mandarin Prawns with Peas

Serves 4

60 ml/4 tbsp groundnut (peanut) oil

1 clove garlic, minced

1 slice ginger root, minced

450 g/1 lb peeled prawns

30 ml/2 tbsp rice wine or dry sherry

225 g/8 oz frozen peas, thawed

30 ml/2 tbsp soy sauce

15 ml/1 tbsp cornflour (cornstarch)

45 ml/3 tbsp water

Heat the oil and fry the garlic and ginger until lightly browned. Add the prawns and stir-fry for 1 minute. Add the wine or sherry and stir together well. Add the peas and stir-fry for 5 minutes. Add the remaining ingredients and stir-fry for 2 minutes.

Peking Prawns

Serves 4

30 ml/2 tbsp groundnut (peanut) oil

2 cloves garlic, crushed

1 slice ginger root, finely chopped

225 g/8 oz peeled prawns

4 spring onions (scallions), thickly sliced

120 ml/4 fl oz/¬Ω cup chicken stock

5 ml/1 tsp brown sugar

5 ml/1 tsp soy sauce

5 ml/1 tsp hoisin sauce

5 ml/1 tsp tabasco sauce

Heat the oil with the garlic and ginger and fry until the garlic is lightly browned. Add the prawns and stir-fry for 1 minute. Add the spring onions and stir-fry for 1 minute. Add the remaining ingredients, bring to the boil, cover and simmer for 4 minutes, stirring occasionally. Check the seasoning and add a little more tabasco sauce if you prefer.

Prawns with Peppers

Serves 4

30 ml/2 tbsp groundnut (peanut) oil

1 green pepper, cut into chunks

450 g/1 lb peeled prawns

10 ml/2 tsp cornflour (cornstarch)

60 ml/4 tbsp water

5 ml/1 tsp rice wine or dry sherry

2.5 ml/¬Ω tsp salt

45 ml/2 tbsp tomato pur√©e (paste)

Heat the oil and stir-fry the pepper for 2 minutes. Add the prawns and tomato pur√©e and stir well. Blend the cornflour water, wine or sherry and salt to a paste, stir it into the pan and simmer, stirring, until the sauce clears and thickens.

Stir-Fried Prawns with Pork

Serves 4

225 g/8 oz peeled prawns

100 g/4 oz lean pork, shredded

60 ml/4 tbsp rice wine or dry sherry

1 egg white

45 ml/3 tbsp cornflour (cornstarch)

5 ml/1 tsp salt

15 ml/1 tbsp water (optional)

90 ml/6 tbsp groundnut (peanut) oil

45 ml/3 tbsp fish stock

5 ml/1 tsp sesame oil

Place the prawns and pork in separate bowls. Mix together 45 ml/ 3 tbsp of wine or sherry, the egg white, 30 ml/2 tbsp of cornflour and the salt to make a loose batter, adding the water if necessary. Divide the mixture between the pork and prawns and stir well to coat them evenly. Heat the oil and fry the pork and prawns for a few minutes until golden brown. Remove from the pan and pour off all but 15 ml/1 tbsp of oil. Add the stock to the pan with the remaining wine or sherry and cornflour. Bring to the boil and simmer, stirring, until the sauce thickens. Pour over the prawns and pork and serve sprinkled with sesame oil.

Deep-Fried Prawns with Sherry Sauce

Serves 4

50 g/2 oz/¬Ω cup plain (all-purpose) flour

2.5 ml/¬Ω tsp salt

1 egg, lightly beaten

30 ml/2 tbsp water

450 g/1 lb peeled prawns

oil for deep-frying

15 ml/1 tbsp groundnut (peanut) oil

1 onion, finely chopped

45 ml/3 tbsp rice wine or dry sherry

15 ml/1 tbsp soy sauce

120 ml/4 fl oz/¬Ω cup fish stock

10 ml/2 tsp cornflour (cornstarch)

30 ml/2 tbsp water

Beat together the flour, salt, egg and water to make a batter, adding a little more water if necessary. Mix with the prawns until they are well coated. Heat the oil and deep-fry the prawns for a few minutes until crispy and golden. Drain on kitchen paper and arrange on a warmed serving dish. Meanwhile, heat the oil and fry the onion until softened. Add the wine or sherry, soy sauce and stock, bring to the boil and simmer for 4 minutes. Mix the cornflour and water to a paste, stir into the pan and simmer, stirring, until the sauce clears and thickens. Pour the sauce over the prawns and serve.

Deep-Fried Sesame Prawns

Serves 4

450 g/1 lb peeled prawns
¬Ω egg white
5 ml/1 tsp soy sauce
5 ml/1 tsp sesame oil
50 g/2 oz/¬Ω cup cornflour (cornstarch)
salt and freshly ground white pepper

oil for deep-frying

60 ml/4 tbsp sesame seeds

lettuce leaves

Mix the prawns with the egg white, soy sauce, sesame oil, cornflour, salt and pepper. Add a little water if the mixture is too thick. Heat the oil and deep-fry the prawns for a few minutes until lightly golden. Meanwhile, toast the sesame seeds briefly in a dry pan until golden. Drain the prawns and mix with the sesame seeds. Serve on a bed of lettuce.

Stir-Fried Prawns in their Shells

Serves 4

60 ml/4 tbsp groundnut (peanut) oil

750 g/1¬Ω lb unpeeled prawns

3 spring onions (scallions), chopped

3 slices ginger root, minced

2.5 ml/¬Ω tsp salt

15 ml/1 tbsp rice wine or dry sherry

120 ml/4 fl oz/¬Ω cup tomato ketchup (catsup)

15 ml/1 tbsp soy sauce

15 ml/1 tbsp sugar

15 ml/1 tbsp cornflour (cornstarch)

60 ml/4 tbsp water

Heat the oil and fry the prawns for 1 minute if cooked or until they turn pink if they are uncooked. Add the spring onions, ginger, salt and wine or sherry and stir-fry for 1 minute. Add the tomato ketchup, soy sauce and sugar and stir-fry for 1 minute. Mix together the cornflour and water, stir it into the pan and simmer, stirring, until the sauce clears and thickens.

Soft-Fried Prawns

Serves 4

75 g/3 oz/heaped ¬° cup cornflour (cornstarch)

1 egg white

5 ml/1 tsp rice wine or dry sherry

salt

350 g/12 oz peeled prawns

oil for deep-frying

Beat together the cornflour, egg white, wine or sherry and a pinch of salt to make a thick batter. Dip the prawns in the batter until they are well coated. Heat the oil until moderately hot and fry the prawns for a few minutes until golden brown. Remove from the oil, reheat it until hot then fry the prawns again until crisp and brown.

Prawn Tempura

Serves 4

450 g/1 lb peeled prawns
30 ml/2 tbsp plain (all-purpose) flour
30 ml/2 tbsp cornflour (cornstarch)
30 ml/2 tbsp water
2 eggs, beaten
oil for deep-frying

Cut the prawns half way through on the inner curve and spread open to make a butterfly. Mix the flour, cornflour and water to a batter then stir in the eggs. Heat the oil and deep-fry the prawns until golden brown.

Sub Gum

Serves 4

30 ml/2 tbsp groundnut (peanut) oil

2 spring onions (scallions), chopped

1 clove garlic, crushed

1 slice ginger root, chopped

100 g/4 oz chicken breast, cut into strips

100 g/4 oz ham, cut into strips

100 g/4 oz bamboo shoots, cut into strips

100 g/4 oz water chestnuts, cut into strips

225 g/8 oz peeled prawns

30 ml/2 tbsp soy sauce

30 ml/2 tbsp rice wine or dry sherry

5 ml/1 tsp salt

5 ml/1 tsp sugar

5 ml/1 tsp cornflour (cornstarch)

Heat the oil and fry the spring onions, garlic and ginger until lightly browned. Add the chicken and stir-fry for 1 minute. Add the ham, bamboo shoots and water chestnuts and stir-fry for 3 minutes. Add the prawns and stir-fry for 1 minute. Add the soy sauce, wine or sherry, salt and sugar and stir-fry for 2 minutes.

Mix the cornflour with a little water, stir it into the pan and simmer, stirring for 2 minutes.

Prawns with Tofu

Serves 4

45 ml/3 tbsp groundnut (peanut) oil

225 g/8 oz tofu, cubed

1 spring onion (scallion), minced

1 clove garlic, crushed

15 ml/1 tbsp soy sauce

5 ml/1 tsp sugar

90 ml/6 tbsp fish stock

225 g/8 oz peeled prawns

15 ml/1 tbsp cornflour (cornstarch)

45 ml/3 tbsp water

Heat half the oil and fry the tofu until lightly browned then remove it from the pan. Heat the remaining oil and stir-fry the spring onions and garlic until lightly browned. Add the soy sauce, sugar and stock and bring to the boil. Add the prawns and stir over a low heat for 3 minutes. Blend the cornflour and water to a paste, stir into the pan and simmer, stirring, until the sauce thickens. Return the tofu to the pan and simmer gently until heated through.

Prawns with Tomatoes

Serves 4

2 egg whites

30 ml/2 tbsp cornflour (cornstarch)

5 ml/1 tsp salt

450 g/1 lb peeled prawns

oil for deep-frying

30 ml/2 tbsp rice wine or dry sherry

225 g/8 oz tomatoes, skinned, seeded and chopped

Mix together the egg whites, cornflour and salt. Stir in the prawns until they are well coated. Heat the oil and deep-fry the prawns until cooked. Pour off all but 15 ml/1 tbsp of the oil and reheat. Add the wine or sherry and tomatoes and bring to the boil. Stir in the prawns and heat through quickly before serving.

Prawns with Tomato Sauce

Serves 4

30 ml/2 tbsp groundnut (peanut) oil

1 clove garlic, crushed

2 slices ginger root, minced

2.5 ml/¬Ω tsp salt

15 ml/1 tbsp rice wine or dry sherry

15 ml/1 tbsp soy sauce

6 ml/4 tbsp tomato ketchup (catsup)

120 ml/4 fl oz/¬Ω cup fish stock

350 g/12 oz peeled prawns

10 ml/2 tsp cornflour (cornstarch)

30 ml/2 tbsp water

Heat the oil and stir-fry the garlic, ginger and salt for 2 minutes. Add the wine or sherry, soy sauce, tomato ketchup and stock and bring to the boil. Add the prawns, cover and simmer for 2 minutes. Mix the cornflour and water to a paste, stir it into the pan and simmer, stirring, until the sauce clears and thickens.

Serves 4

60 ml/4 tbsp groundnut (peanut) oil

15 ml/1 tbsp minced ginger

15 ml/1 tbsp minced garlic

15 ml/1 tbsp minced spring onion

60 ml/4 tbsp tomato purée (paste)

15 ml/1 tbsp chilli sauce

450 g/1 lb peeled prawns

15 ml/1 tbsp cornflour (cornstarch)

15 ml/1 tbsp water

Heat the oil and stir-fry the ginger, garlic and spring onion for 1 minute. Add the tomato purée and chilli sauce and mix well. Add the prawns and stir-fry for 2 minutes. Blend the cornflour and water to a paste, stir it into the pan and simmer until the sauce thickens. Serve at once.

Deep-Fried Prawns with Tomato Sauce

Serves 4

50 g/2 oz/¬Ω cup plain (all-purpose) flour

2.5 ml/¬Ω tsp salt

1 egg, lightly beaten

30 ml/2 tbsp water

450 g/1 lb peeled prawns

oil for deep-frying

30 ml/2 tbsp groundnut (peanut) oil

1 onion, finely chopped

2 slices ginger root, minced

75 ml/5 tbsp tomato ketchup (catsup)

10 ml/2 tsp cornflour (cornstarch)

30 ml/2 tbsp water

Beat together the flour, salt, egg and water to make a batter, adding a little more water if necessary. Mix with the prawns until they are well coated. Heat the oil and deep-fry the prawns for a few minutes until crispy and golden. Drain on kitchen paper.

Meanwhile heat the oil and fry the onion and ginger until softened. Add the tomato ketchup and simmer for 3 minutes. Mix the cornflour and water to a paste, stir into the pan and simmer, stirring, until the sauce thickens. Add the prawns to the pan and simmer until heated through. Serve at once.

Prawns with Vegetables

Serves 4

15 ml/1 tbsp groundnut (peanut) oil

225 g/8 oz broccoli florets

225 g/8 oz button mushrooms

225 g/8 oz bamboo shoots, sliced

450 g/1 lb peeled prawns

120 ml/4 fl oz/¬Ω cup chicken stock

5 ml/1 tsp cornflour (cornstarch)

5 ml/1 tsp oyster sauce

2.5 ml/¬Ω tsp sugar

2.5 ml/¬Ω tsp grated ginger root

pinch of freshly ground pepper

Heat the oil and stir-fry the broccoli for 1 minute. Add the mushrooms and bamboo shoots and stir-fry for 2 minutes. Add the prawns and stir-fry for 2 minutes. Mix together the remaining ingredients and stir into the prawn mixture. Bring to the boil, stirring, then simmer for 1 minute, stirring continuously.

Prawns with Water Chestnuts

Serves 4

60 ml/4 tbsp groundnut (peanut) oil

1 clove garlic, minced

1 slice ginger root, minced

450 g/1 lb peeled prawns

30 ml/2 tbsp rice wine or dry sherry 225 g/8 oz water chestnuts, sliced

30 ml/2 tbsp soy sauce

15 ml/1 tbsp cornflour (cornstarch)

45 ml/3 tbsp water

Heat the oil and fry the garlic and ginger until lightly browned. Add the prawns and stir-fry for 1 minute. Add the wine or sherry and stir together well. Add the water chestnuts and stir-fry for 5 minutes. Add the remaining ingredients and stir-fry for 2 minutes.

Prawn Wontons

Serves 4

450 g/1 lb peeled prawns, chopped
225 g/8 oz mixed vegetables, chopped
15 ml/1 tbsp soy sauce
2.5 ml/¬Ω tsp salt
few drops of sesame oil
40 wonton skins
oil for deep-frying

Mix together the prawns, vegetables, soy sauce, salt and sesame oil.

To fold the wontons, hold the skin in the palm of your left hand and spoon a little filling into the centre. Moisten the edges with egg and fold the skin into a triangle, sealing the edges. Moisten the corners with egg and twist them together.

Heat the oil and fry the wontons a few at a time until golden brown. Drain well before serving.

Abalone with Chicken

Serves 4

400 g/14 oz canned abalone

30 ml/2 tbsp groundnut (peanut) oil

100 g/4 oz chicken breast, diced

100 g/4 oz bamboo shoots, sliced

250 ml/8 fl oz/1 cup fish stock

15 ml/1 tbsp rice wine or dry sherry

5 ml/1 tsp sugar

2.5 ml/¬Ω tsp salt

15 ml/1 tbsp cornflour (cornstarch)

45 ml/3 tbsp water

Drain and slice the abalone, reserving the juice. Heat the oil and stir-fry the chicken until lightly coloured. Add the abalone and bamboo shoots and stir-fry for 1 minute. Add the abalone liquid, stock, wine or sherry, sugar and salt, bring to the boil and simmer for 2 minutes. Mix the cornflour and water to a paste and simmer, stirring, until the sauce clears and thickens. Serve at once.

Abalone with Asparagus

Serves 4

10 dried Chinese mushrooms

30 ml/2 tbsp groundnut (peanut) oil

15 ml/1 tbsp water

225 g/8 oz asparagus

2.5 ml/½ tsp fish sauce

15 ml/1 tbsp cornflour (cornstarch)

225 g/8 oz canned abalone, sliced

60 ml/4 tbsp stock

½ small carrot, sliced

5 ml/1 tsp soy sauce

5 ml/1 tsp oyster sauce

5 ml/1 tsp rice wine or dry sherry

Soak the mushrooms in warm water for 30 minutes then drain. Discard the stalks. Heat 15 ml/1 tbsp of oil with the water and fry the mushroom caps for 10 minutes. Meanwhile, cook the asparagus in boiling water with the fish sauce and 5 ml/1 tsp cornflour until tender. Drain well and arrange on a warmed serving plate with the mushrooms. Keep them warm. Heat the remaining oil and fry the abalone for a few seconds then add the stock, carrot, soy sauce, oyster sauce, wine or sherry and remaining cornflour. Cook for about 5 minutes until well done then spoon over the asparagus and serve.

Abalone with Mushrooms

Serves 4

6 dried Chinese mushrooms

400 g/14 oz canned abalone

45 ml/3 tbsp groundnut (peanut) oil

2.5 ml/¬Ω tsp salt

15 ml/1 tbsp rice wine or dry sherry

3 spring onions (scallions), thickly sliced

Soak the mushrooms in warm water for 30 minutes then drain. Discard the stalks and slice the caps. Drain and slice the abalone, reserving the juice. Heat the oil and stir-fry the salt and mushrooms for 2 minutes. Add the abalone liquid and sherry, bring to the boil, cover and simmer for 3 minutes. Add the abalone and spring onions and simmer until heated through. Serve at once.

Abalone with Oyster Sauce

Serves 4

400 g/14 oz canned abalone
15 ml/1 tbsp cornflour (cornstarch)
15 ml/1 tbsp soy sauce
45 ml/3 tbsp oyster sauce
30 ml/2 tbsp groundnut (peanut) oil
50 g/2 oz smoked ham, minced

Drain the can of abalone and reserve 90 ml/6 tbsp of the liquid. Mix this with the cornflour, soy sauce and oyster sauce. Heat the oil and stir-fry the drained abalone for 1 minute. Stir in the sauce mixture and simmer, stirring, for about 1 minute until heated through. Transfer to a warmed serving plate and serve garnished with ham.

Steamed Clams

Serves 4

24 clams

Scrub the clams thoroughly then soak them in salted water for a few hours. Rinse under running water and arrange on a shallow ovenproof plate. Place on a rack in a steamer, cover and steam over gently simmering water for about 10 minutes until all the clams have opened. Discard any that remain closed. Serve with dips.

Clams with Bean Sprouts

Serves 4

24 clams

15 ml/1 tbsp groundnut (peanut) oil

150 g/5 oz bean sprouts

1 green pepper, cut into strips

2 spring onions (scallions), chopped

15 ml/1 tbsp rice wine or dry sherry

salt and freshly ground pepper

2.5 ml/¬Ω tsp sesame oil

50 g/2 oz smoked ham, chopped

Scrub the clams thoroughly then soak them in salted water for a few hours. Rinse under running water. Bring a pan of water to the boil, add the clams and simmer for a few minutes until they open. Drain and discard any that remain closed. Remove the clams from the shells.

Heat the oil and fry the bean sprouts for 1 minute. Add the pepper and spring onions and stir-fry for 2 minutes. Add the wine or sherry and season with salt and pepper. Heat through then stir in the clams and stir until well mixed and heated through. Transfer to a warmed serving plate and serve sprinkled with sesame oil and ham.

Serves 4

24 clams

15 ml/1 tbsp groundnut (peanut) oil

2 slices ginger root, minced

2 cloves garlic, crushed

15 ml/1 tbsp water

5 ml/1 tsp sesame oil

salt and freshly ground pepper

Scrub the clams thoroughly then soak them in salted water for a few hours. Rinse under running water. Heat the oil and fry the ginger and garlic for 30 seconds. Add the clams, water and sesame oil, cover and cook for about 5 minutes until the clams open. Discard any that remain closed. Season lightly with salt and pepper and serve at once.

Serves 4

24 clams

60 ml/4 tbsp groundnut (peanut) oil

4 cloves garlic, minced

1 onion, minced

2.5 ml/¬Ω tsp salt

Scrub the clams thoroughly then soak them in salted water for a few hours. Rinse under running water then pat dry. Heat the oil and fry the garlic, onion and salt until softened. Add the clams, cover and cook over a low heat for about 5 minutes until all the shells have opened. Discard any that remain closed. Stir-fry gently for a further 1 minute, basting with oil.

Crab Cakes

Serves 4

225 g/8 oz bean sprouts

60 ml/4 tbsp groundnut (peanut) oil 100 g/4 oz bamboo shoots,

cut into strips

1 onion, chopped

225 g/8 oz crab meat, flaked

4 eggs, lightly beaten

15 ml/1 tbsp cornflour (cornstarch)

30 ml/2 tbsp soy sauce

salt and freshly ground pepper

Blanch the bean sprouts in boiling water for 4 minutes then drain. Heat half the oil and stir-fry the bean sprouts, bamboo shoots and onion until softened. Remove from the heat and mix in the remaining ingredients, except the oil. Heat the remaining oil in a clean pan and fry spoonfuls of the crab meat mixture to make small cakes. Fry until lightly browned on both sides then serve at once.

Crab Custard

Serves 4

225 g/8 oz crab meat

5 eggs, beaten

1 spring onion (scallion) finely chopped

250 ml/8 fl oz/1 cup water

5 ml/1 tsp salt

5 ml/1 tsp sesame oil

Mix all the ingredients together well. Place in a bowl, cover and stand in the top of the double boiler over hot water or on a steamer rack. Steam for about 35 minutes until the consistency of custard, stirring occasionally. Serve with rice.

Serves 4

450 g/1 lb Chinese leaves, shredded

45 ml/3 tbsp vegetable oil

2 spring onions (scallions), chopped

225 g/8 oz crab meat

15 ml/1 tbsp soy sauce

15 ml/1 tbsp rice wine or dry sherry

5 ml/1 tsp salt

Blanch the Chinese leaves in boiling water for 2 minutes then drain thoroughly and rinse in cold water. Heat the oil and fry the spring onions until lightly browned. Add the crab meat and stir-fry for 2 minutes. Add the Chinese leaves and stir-fry for 4 minutes. Add the soy sauce, wine or sherry and salt and mix well. Add the stock and cornflour, bring to the boil and simmer, stirring, for 2 minutes until the sauce clears and thickens.

Crab Foo Yung with Bean Sprouts

Serves 4

6 eggs, beaten

45 ml/3 tbsp cornflour (cornstarch)

225 g/8 oz crab meat

100 g/4 oz bean sprouts

2 spring onions (scallions), finely chopped

2.5 ml/¬Ω tsp salt

45 ml/3 tbsp groundnut (peanut) oil

Beat the eggs then beat in the cornflour. Mix in the remaining ingredients except the oil. Heat the oil and pour the mixture into the pan a little at a time to make small pancakes about 7.5 cm/3 in across. Fry until browned on the bottom then turn and brown the other side.

Serves 4

15 ml/1 tbsp groundnut (peanut) oil

2 slices ginger root, chopped

4 spring onions (scallions), chopped

3 cloves garlic, crushed

1 red chilli pepper, chopped

350 g/12 oz crab meat, flaked

2.5 ml/¬Ω tsp fish paste

2.5 ml/¬Ω tsp sesame oil

15 ml/1 tbsp rice wine or dry sherry

5 ml/1 tsp cornflour (cornstarch)

15 ml/1 tbsp water

Heat the oil and fry the ginger, spring onions, garlic and chilli for 2 minutes. Add the crab meat and stir until well coated with the spices. Stir in the fish paste. Mix the remaining ingredients to a paste then stir them into the pan and stir-fry for 1 minutes. Serve at once.

Crab Lo Mein

Serves 4

100 g/4 oz bean sprouts

30 ml/2 tbsp groundnut (peanut) oil

5 ml/1 tsp salt

1 onion, sliced

100 g/4 oz mushrooms, sliced

225 g/8 oz crab meat, flaked

100 g/4 oz bamboo shoots, sliced

Tossed Noodles

30 ml/2 tbsp soy sauce

5 ml/1 tsp sugar

5 ml/1 tsp sesame oil

salt and freshly ground pepper

Blanch the bean sprouts in boiling water for 5 minutes then drain. Heat the oil and fry the salt and onion until softened. Add the mushrooms and stir-fry until softened. Add the crab meat and stir-fry for 2 minutes. Add the bean sprouts and bamboo shoots and stir-fry for 1 minute. Add the drained noodles to the pan and stir gently. Mix the soy sauce, sugar and sesame oil and season with salt and pepper. Stir into the pan until heated through.

Stir-Fried Crab with Pork

Serves 4

30 ml/2 tbsp groundnut (peanut) oil

100 g/4 oz minced (ground) pork

350 g/12 oz crab meat, flaked

2 slices ginger root, minced

2 eggs, lightly beaten

15 ml/1 tbsp soy sauce

15 ml/1 tbsp rice wine or dry sherry

30 ml/2 tbsp water

salt and freshly ground pepper

4 spring onions (scallions), cut into strips

Heat the oil and stir-fry the pork until lightly coloured. Add the crab meat and ginger and stir-fry for 1 minute. Stir in the eggs. Add the soy sauce, wine or sherry, water, salt and pepper and simmer for about 4 minutes, stirring. Serve garnished with spring onions.

Stir-Fried Crab Meat

Serves 4

30 ml/2 tbsp groundnut (peanut) oil

450 g/1 lb crab meat, flaked

2 spring onions (scallions), minced

2 slices ginger root, minced

30 ml/2 tbsp soy sauce

30 ml/2 tbsp rice wine or dry sherry

2.5 ml/¬Ω tsp salt

15 ml/1 tbsp cornflour (cornstarch)

60 ml/4 tbsp water

Heat the oil and stir-fry the crab meat, spring onions and ginger for 1 minute. Add the soy sauce, wine or sherry and salt, cover and simmer for 3 minutes. Mix the cornflour and water to a paste, stir into the pan and simmer, stirring, until the sauce clears and thickens.

Deep-Fried Cuttlefish Balls

Serves 4

450 g/1 lb cuttlefish

50 g/2 oz lard, mashed

1 egg white

2.5 ml/¬Ω tsp sugar

2.5 ml/¬Ω tsp cornflour (cornstarch)

salt and freshly ground pepper

oil for deep-frying

Trim the cuttlefish and mash or pur√©e it to a pulp. Mix with the lard, egg white, sugar and cornflour and season with salt and pepper. Press the mixture into small balls. Heat the oil and fry the cuttlefish balls, in batches if necessary, until they float to the top of the oil and turn golden brown. Drain well and serve at once.

Lobster Cantonese

Serves 4

2 lobsters

30 ml/2 tbsp oil

15 ml/1 tbsp black bean sauce

1 clove garlic, crushed

1 onion, chopped

225 g/8 oz minced (ground) pork

45 ml/3 tbsp soy sauce

5 ml/1 tsp sugar

salt and freshly ground pepper

15 ml/1 tbsp cornflour (cornstarch)

75 ml/5 tbsp water

1 egg, beaten

Break open the lobsters, take out the meat and cut it into 2.5 cm/1 in cubes. Heat the oil and fry the black bean sauce, garlic and onion until lightly browned. Add the pork and fry until browned. Add the soy sauce, sugar, salt, pepper and lobster, cover and simmer for about 10 minutes. Blend the cornflour and water to a paste, stir it into the pan and simmer, stirring, until the sauce clears and thickens. Turn off the heat and stir in the egg before serving.

Deep-Fried Lobster

Serves 4

450 g/1 lb lobster meat

30 ml/2 tbsp soy sauce

5 ml/1 tsp sugar

1 egg, beaten

30 ml/3 tbsp plain (all-purpose) flour

oil for deep-frying

Cut the lobster meat into 2.5 cm/1 in cubes and toss with the soy sauce and sugar. Leave to stand for 15 minutes then drain. Beat the egg and flour then add the lobster and toss well to coat. Heat the oil and deep-fry the lobster until golden brown. Drain on kitchen paper before serving.

Serves 4

4 eggs, lightly beaten
60 ml/4 tbsp water
5 ml/1 tsp salt
15 ml/1 tbsp soy sauce
450 g/1 lb lobster meat, flaked
15 ml/1 tbsp chopped smoked ham
15 ml/1 tbsp chopped fresh parsley

Beat the eggs with the water, salt and soy sauce. Pour into an ovenproof bowl and sprinkle with lobster meat. Place the bowl on a rack in a steamer, cover and steam for 20 minutes until the eggs are set. Serve garnished with ham and parsley.

Lobster with Mushrooms

Serves 4

450 g/1 lb lobster meat

15 ml/1 tbsp cornflour (cornstarch)

60 ml/4 tbsp water

30 ml/2 tbsp groundnut (peanut) oil

4 spring onions (scallions), thickly sliced

100 g/4 oz mushrooms, sliced

2.5 ml/¬Ω tsp salt

1 clove garlic, crushed

30 ml/2 tbsp soy sauce

15 ml/1 tbsp rice wine or dry sherry

Cut the lobster meat into 2.5 cm/1 in cubes. Mix the cornflour and water to a paste and toss the lobster cubes in the mixture to coat. Heat half the oil and fry the lobster cubes until lightly browned them remove them from the pan. Heat the remaining oil and fry the spring onions until lightly browned. Add the mushrooms and stir-fry for 3 minutes. Add the salt, garlic, soy sauce and wine or sherry and stir-fry for 2 minutes. Return the lobster to the pan and stir-fry until heated through.

Lobster Tails with Pork

Serves 4

3 dried Chinese mushrooms

4 lobster tails

60 ml/4 tbsp groundnut (peanut) oil

100 g/4 oz minced (ground) pork

50 g/2 oz water chestnuts, finely chopped

salt and freshly ground pepper

2 cloves garlic, crushed

45 ml/3 tbsp soy sauce

30 ml/2 tbsp rice wine or dry sherry

30 ml/2 tbsp black bean sauce

10 ml/2 tbsp cornflour (cornstarch)

120 ml/4 fl oz/¬Ω cup water

Soak the mushrooms in warm water for 30 minutes then drain. Discard the stalks and chop the caps. Cut the lobster tails in half lengthways. Remove the meat from the lobster tails, reserving the shells. Heat half the oil and fry the pork until lightly coloured. Remove from the heat and mix in the mushrooms, lobster meat, water chestnuts, salt and pepper. Press the meat back into the lobster shells and arrange on an ovenproof plate. Place on a rack in a steamer, cover and steam for about 20 minutes until cooked.

Meanwhile, heat the remaining oil and fry the garlic, soy sauce, wine or sherry and black bean sauce for 2 minutes. Mix the cornflour and water to a paste, stir it into the pan and simmer, stirring, until the sauce thickens. Arrange the lobster on a warmed serving plate, pour over the sauce and serve at once.

Stir-Fried Lobster

Serves 4

450 g/1 lb lobster tails

30 ml/2 tbsp groundnut (peanut) oil

1 clove garlic, crushed

2.5 ml/¬Ω tsp salt

350 g/12 oz bean sprouts

50 g/2 oz button mushrooms

4 spring onions (scallions), thickly sliced

150 ml/¬° pt/generous ¬Ω cup chicken stock

15 ml/1 tbsp cornflour (cornstarch)

Bring a pan of water to the boil, add the lobster tails and boil for 1 minute. Drain, cool, remove the shell and cut into thick slices. Heat the oil with the garlic and salt and fry until the garlic is lightly browned. Add the lobster and stir-fry for 1 minute. Add the bean sprouts and mushrooms and stir-fry for 1 minute. Stir in the spring onions. Add most of the stock, bring to the boil, cover and simmer for 3 minutes. Mix the cornflour with the remaining stock, stir it into the pan and simmer, stirring, until the sauce clears and thickens.

Lobster Nests

Serves 4

30 ml/2 tbsp groundnut (peanut) oil

5 ml/1 tsp salt

1 onion, thinly sliced

100 g/4 oz mushrooms, sliced

100 g/4 oz bamboo shoots, sliced 225 g/8 oz cooked lobster meat

15 ml/1 tbsp rice wine or dry sherry

120 ml/4 fl oz/¬Ω cup chicken stock

pinch of freshly ground pepper

10 ml/2 tsp cornflour (cornstarch)

15 ml/1 tbsp water

4 noodle baskets

Heat the oil and fry the salt and onion until softened. Add the mushrooms and bamboo shoots and stir-fry for 2 minutes. Add the lobster meat, wine or sherry and stock, bring to the boil, cover and simmer for 2 minutes. Season with pepper. Mix the cornflour and water to a paste, stir into the pan and simmer, stirring, until the sauce thickens. Arrange the noodle nests on a warmed serving plate and top with the lobster stir-fry.

Serves 4

45 ml/3 tbsp groundnut (peanut) oil

2 cloves garlic, crushed

2 slices ginger root, minced

30 ml/2 tbsp black bean sauce

15 ml/1 tbsp soy sauce

1.5 kg/3 lb mussels, scrubbed and bearded

2 spring onions (scallions), chopped

Heat the oil and fry the garlic and ginger for 30 seconds. Add the black bean sauce and soy sauce and fry for 10 seconds. Add the mussels, cover and cook for about 6 minutes until the mussels have opened. Discard any that remain closed. Transfer to a warmed serving dish and serve sprinkled with spring onions.

Serves 4

45 ml/3 tbsp groundnut (peanut) oil

2 cloves garlic, crushed

4 slices ginger root, minced

1.5 kg/3 lb mussels, scrubbed and bearded

45 ml/3 tbsp water

15 ml/1 tbsp oyster sauce

Heat the oil and fry the garlic and ginger for 30 seconds. Add the mussels and water, cover and cook for about 6 minutes until the mussels have opened. Discard any that remain closed. Transfer to a warmed serving dish and serve sprinkled with oyster sauce.

Serves 4

1.5 kg/3 lb mussels, scrubbed and bearded

45 ml/3 tbsp soy sauce

3 spring onions (scallions), finely chopped

Arrange the mussels on a rack in a steamer, cover and steam over boiling water for about 10 minutes until all the mussels have opened. Discard any that remain closed. Transfer to a warmed serving dish and serve sprinkled with soy sauce and spring onions.

Deep-Fried Oysters

Serves 4

24 oysters, shelled

salt and freshly ground pepper

1 egg, beaten

50 g/2 oz/¬Ω cup plain (all-purpose) flour

250 ml/8 fl oz/1 cup water

oil for deep-frying

4 spring onions (scallions), chopped

Sprinkle the oysters with salt and pepper. Beat the egg with the flour and water to a batter and use to coat the oysters. Heat the oil and deep-fry the oysters until golden brown. Drain on kitchen paper and serve garnished with spring onions.

Oysters with Bacon

Serves 4

175 g/6 oz bacon

24 oysters, shelled

1 egg, lightly beaten

15 ml/1 tbsp water

45 ml/3 tbsp groundnut (peanut) oil

2 onions, chopped

15 ml/1 tbsp cornflour (cornstarch)

15 ml/1 tbsp soy sauce

90 ml/6 tbsp chicken stock

Cut the bacon into pieces and wrap one piece around each oyster. Beat the egg with the water then dip in the oysters to coat. Heat half the oil and fry the oysters until lightly browned on both sides then remove them from the pan and drain off the fat. Heat the remaining oil and fry the onions until softened. Mix the cornflour, soy sauce and stock to a paste, pour into the pan and simmer, stirring, until the sauce clears and thickens. Pour over the oysters and serve at once.

Deep-Fried Oysters with Ginger

Serves 4

24 oysters, shelled

2 slices ginger root, minced

30 ml/2 tbsp soy sauce

15 ml/1 tbsp rice wine or dry sherry

4 spring onions (scallions), cut into strips

100 g/4 oz bacon

1 egg

50 g/2 oz/¬Ω cup plain (all-purpose) flour

salt and freshly ground pepper

oil for deep-frying

1 lemon, cut into wedges

Place the oysters in a bowl with the ginger, soy sauce and wine or sherry and toss well to coat. Leave to stand for 30 minutes. Place a few strips of spring onion on top of each oyster. Cut the bacon into pieces and wrap a piece around each oyster. Beat the egg and flour to a batter and season with salt and pepper. Dip the oysters in the batter until well coated. Heat the oil and deep-fry the oysters until golden brown. Serve garnished with lemon wedges.

Oysters with Black Bean Sauce

Serves 4

350 g/12 oz shelled oysters

120 ml/4 fl oz/¬Ω cup groundnut (peanut) oil

2 cloves garlic, crushed

3 spring onions (scallions), sliced

15 ml/1 tbsp black bean sauce

30 ml/2 tbsp dark soy sauce

15 ml/1 tbsp sesame oil

pinch chilli powder

Blanch the oysters in boiling water for 30 seconds then drain. Heat the oil and stir-fry the garlic and spring onions for 30 seconds. Add the black bean sauce, soy sauce, sesame oil and oysters and season to taste with chilli powder. Stir-fry until heated through and serve at once.

Scallops with Bamboo Shoots

Serves 4

60 ml/4 tbsp groundnut (peanut) oil

6 spring onions (scallions), chopped

225 g/8 oz mushrooms, quartered

15 ml/1 tbsp sugar

450 g/1 lb shelled scallops

2 slices ginger root, chopped

225 g/8 oz bamboo shoots, sliced

salt and freshly ground pepper

300 ml/¬Ω pt/1 ¬° cups water

30 ml/2 tbsp wine vinegar

30 ml/2 tbsp cornflour (cornstarch)

150 ml/¬° pt/generous ¬Ω cup water

45 ml/3 tbsp soy sauce

Heat the oil and fry the spring onions and mushrooms for 2 minutes. Add the sugar, scallops, ginger, bamboo shoots, salt and pepper, cover and cook for 5 minutes. Add the water and wine vinegar, bring to the boil, cover and simmer for 5 minutes. Blend the cornflour and water to a paste, stir into the pan and simmer, stirring, until the sauce thickens. Season with soy sauce and serve.

Scallops with Egg

Serves 4

45 ml/3 tbsp groundnut (peanut) oil

350 g/12 oz shelled scallops

25 g/1 oz smoked ham, chopped

30 ml/2 tbsp rice wine or dry sherry

5 ml/1 tsp sugar

2.5 ml/¬Ω tsp salt

pinch of freshly ground pepper

2 eggs, lightly beaten

15 ml/1 tbsp soy sauce

Heat the oil and stir-fry the scallops for 30 seconds. Add the ham and stir-fry for 1 minute. Add the wine or sherry, sugar, salt and pepper and stir-fry for 1 minute. Add the eggs and stir gently over a high heat until the ingredients are well coated in egg. Serve sprinkled with soy sauce.

Serves 4

350 g/12 oz scallops, sliced

3 slices ginger root, minced

¬Ω small carrot, sliced

1 clove garlic, crushed

45 ml/3 tbsp plain (all-purpose) flour

2.5 ml/¬Ω tsp bicarbonate of soda (baking soda)

30 ml/2 tbsp groundnut (peanut) oil

15 ml/1 tbsp water

1 banana, sliced

oil for deep-frying

275 g/10 oz broccoli

salt

5 ml/1 tsp sesame oil

2.5 ml/¬Ω tsp chilli sauce

2.5 ml/¬Ω tsp wine vinegar

2.5 ml/¬Ω tsp tomato pur√©e (paste)

Mix the scallops with the ginger, carrot and garlic and leave to stand. Mix the flour, bicarbonate of soda, 15 ml/ 1 tbsp of oil and the water to a paste and use to coat the banana slices. Heat the oil and deep-fry the banana until golden brown then drain and arrange around a warmed serving plate. Meanwhile, cook the broccoli in boiling, salted water until just tender then drain. Heat the remaining oil with the sesame oil and stir-fry the broccoli briefly then arrange it round the plate with the bananas. Add the chilli sauce, wine vinegar and tomato purée to the pan and stir-fry the scallops until just cooked. Spoon on to the serving plate and serve at once.

Scallops with Ginger

Serves 4

45 ml/3 tbsp groundnut (peanut) oil

2.5 ml/¬Ω tsp salt

3 slices ginger root, minced

2 spring onions (scallions), thickly sliced

450 g/1 lb shelled scallops, halved

15 ml/1 tbsp cornflour (cornstarch)

60 ml/4 tbsp water

Heat the oil and fry the salt and ginger for 30 seconds. Add the spring onions and stir-fry until lightly browned. Add the scallops and stir-fry for 3 minutes. Mix the cornflour and water to a paste, add to the pan and simmer, stirring, until thickened. Serve at once.

Serves 4

450 g/1 lb shelled scallops, halved
250 ml/8 fl oz/1 cup rice wine or dry sherry
1 onion, finely chopped
2 slices ginger root, minced
2.5 ml/¬Ω tsp salt
100 g/4 oz smoked ham, chopped

Place the scallops in a bowl and add the wine or sherry. Cover and leave to marinate for 30 minutes, turning occasionally, then drain the scallops and discard the marinade. Place the scallops in an ovenproof dish with the remaining ingredients. Place the dish on a rack in a steamer, cover and steam over boiling water for about 6 minutes until the scallops are tender.

Serves 4

225 g/8 oz shelled scallops

30 ml/2 tbsp chopped fresh coriander

4 eggs, beaten

15 ml/1 tbsp rice wine or dry sherry

salt and freshly ground pepper

15 ml/1 tbsp groundnut (peanut) oil

Place the scallops in a steamer and steam for about 3 minutes until cooked, depending on the size. Remove from the steamer and sprinkle with coriander. Beat the eggs with the wine or sherry and season to taste with salt and pepper. Mix in the scallops and coriander. Heat the oil and fry the egg and scallop mixture, stirring constantly, until the eggs are just set. Serve immediately.

Serves 4

45 ml/3 tbsp groundnut (peanut) oil
1 onion, sliced
450 g/1 lb shelled scallops, quartered
salt and freshly ground pepper
15 ml/1 tbsp rice wine or dry sherry

Heat the oil and fry the onion until softened. Add the scallops and stir-fry until lightly browned. Season with salt and pepper, sprinkle with wine or sherry and serve at once.

Scallops with Vegetables

Serves 4,Äì6

4 dried Chinese mushrooms

2 onions

30 ml/2 tbsp groundnut (peanut) oil

3 stalks celery, diagonally sliced

225 g/8 oz green beans, diagonally sliced

10 ml/2 tsp grated ginger root

1 clove garlic, crushed

20 ml/4 tsp cornflour (cornstarch)

250 ml/8 fl oz/1 cup chicken stock

30 ml/2 tbsp rice wine or dry sherry

30 ml/2 tbsp soy sauce

450 g/1 lb shelled scallops, quartered

6 spring onions (scallions), sliced

425 g/15 oz canned baby corn cobs

Soak the mushrooms in warm water for 30 minutes then drain. Discard the stalks and slice the caps. Cut the onions into wedges and separate the layers. Heat the oil and stir-fry the onions, celery, beans, ginger and garlic for 3 minutes. Blend the cornflour with a little of the stock then mix in the remaining stock, wine or sherry and soy sauce. Add to the wok and bring to the boil, stirring. Add the mushrooms, scallops, spring onions and corn and stir-fry for about 5 minutes until the scallops are tender.

Scallops with Peppers

Serves 4

30 ml/2 tbsp groundnut (peanut) oil

3 spring onions (scallions), chopped

1 clove garlic, crushed

2 slices ginger root, chopped

2 red peppers, diced

450 g/1 lb shelled scallops

30 ml/2 tbsp rice wine or dry sherry

15 ml/1 tbsp soy sauce

15 ml/1 tbsp yellow bean sauce

5 ml/1 tsp sugar

5 ml/1 tsp sesame oil

Heat the oil and stir-fry the spring onions, garlic and ginger for 30 seconds. Add the peppers and stir-fry for 1 minute. Add the scallops and stir-fry for 30 seconds then add the remaining ingredients and cook for about 3 minutes until the scallops are tender.

Squid with Bean Sprouts

Serves 4

450 g/1 lb squid

30 ml/2 tbsp groundnut (peanut) oil

15 ml/1 tbsp rice wine or dry sherry

100 g/4 oz bean sprouts

15 ml/1 tbsp soy sauce

salt

1 red chilli pepper, shredded

2 slices ginger root, shredded

2 spring onions (scallions), shredded

Remove the head, guts and membrane from the squid and cut into large pieces. Cut a criss-cross pattern on each piece. Bring a pan of water to the boil, add the squid and simmer until the pieces roll up then remove and drain. Heat half the oil and stir-fry the squid quickly. Sprinkle with wine or sherry. Meanwhile, heat the remaining oil and stir-fry the bean sprouts until just tender. Season with soy sauce and salt. Arrange the chilli pepper, ginger and spring onions around a serving plate. Pile the bean sprouts in the centre and top with the squid. Serve at once.

Deep-Fried Squid

Serves 4

50 g/2 oz plain (all-purpose) flour
25 g/1 oz/¬° cup cornflour (cornstarch)
2.5 ml/¬Ω tsp baking powder
2.5 ml/¬Ω tsp salt
1 egg
75 ml/5 tbsp water
15 ml/1 tbsp groundnut (peanut) oil

450 g/1 lb squid, cut into rings

oil for deep-frying

Beat the flour, cornflour, baking powder, salt, egg, water and oil together to make a batter. Dip the squid in the batter until well coated. Heat the oil and deep-fry the squid a few pieces at a time until golden brown. Drain on kitchen paper before serving.

Squid Parcels

Serves 4

8 dried Chinese mushrooms

450 g/1 lb squid

100 g/4 oz smoked ham

100 g/4 oz tofu

1 egg, beaten

15 ml/1 tbsp plain (all-purpose) flour

2.5 ml/¬Ω tsp sugar

2.5 ml/¬Ω tsp sesame oil

salt and freshly ground pepper

8 wonton skins

oil for deep-frying

Soak the mushrooms in warm water for 30 minutes then drain. Discard the stalks. Trim the squid and cut into 8 pieces. Cut the ham and tofu into 8 pieces. Place them all in a bowl. Mix the egg with the flour, sugar, sesame oil, salt and pepper. Pour over the ingredients in the bowl and mix together gently. Arrange a mushroom cap and a piece each of squid, ham and tofu just below the centre of each wonton skin. Fold up the bottom corner, fold in the sides then roll up, moistening the edges with water to seal. Heat the oil and deep-fry the parcels for about 8 minutes until golden brown. Drain well before serving.

Fried Squid Rolls

Serves 4

45 ml/3 tbsp groundnut (peanut) oil

225 g/8 oz squid rings

1 large green pepper, cut into chunks

100 g/4 oz bamboo shoots, sliced

2 spring onions (scallions), finely chopped

1 slice ginger root, finely chopped

45 ml/2 tbsp soy sauce

30 ml/2 tbsp rice wine or dry sherry

15 ml/1 tbsp cornflour (cornstarch)

15 ml/1 tbsp fish stock or water

5 ml/1 tsp sugar

5 ml/1 tsp wine vinegar

5 ml/1 tsp sesame oil

salt and freshly ground pepper

Heat 15 ml/1 tbsp oil and fry the squid rings quickly until just sealed. Meanwhile, heat the remaining oil in a separate pan and stir-fry the pepper, bamboo shoots, spring onions and ginger for 2 minutes. Add the squid and stir-fry for 1 minute. Stir in the soy sauce, wine or sherry, cornflour, stock, sugar, wine vinegar and sesame oil and season with salt and pepper. Stir-fry until the sauce clears and thickens.

Squid Stir-Fry

Serves 4

45 ml/3 tbsp groundnut (peanut) oil

3 spring onions (scallions), thickly sliced

2 slices ginger root, minced

450 g/1 lb squid, cut into chunks

15 ml/1 tbsp soy sauce

15 ml/1 tbsp rice wine or dry sherry

5 ml/1 tsp cornflour (cornstarch)

15 ml/1 tbsp water

Heat the oil and fry the spring onions and ginger until softened. Add the squid and stir-fry until coated in oil. Add the soy sauce and wine or sherry, cover and simmer for 2 minutes. Mix the cornflour and water to a paste, add it to the pan and simmer, stirring, until the sauce thickens and the squid is tender.

Squid with Dried Mushrooms

Serves 4

50 g/2 oz dried Chinese mushrooms

450 g/1 lb squid rings

45 ml/3 tbsp groundnut (peanut) oil

45 ml/3 tbsp soy sauce

2 spring onions (scallions), finely chopped

1 slice ginger root, minced

225 g/8 oz bamboo shoots, cut into strips

30 ml/2 tbsp cornflour (cornstarch)

150 ml/¬° pt/generous ¬Ω cup fish stock

Soak the mushrooms in warm water for 30 minutes then drain. Discard the stems and slice the caps. Blanch the squid rings for a few seconds in boiling water. Heat the oil then stir in the mushrooms, soy sauce, spring onions and ginger and stir-fry for 2 minutes. Add the squid and bamboo shoots and stir-fry for 2 minutes. Mix together the cornflour and stock and stir it into the pan. Simmer, stirring, until the sauce clears and thickens.

Squid with Vegetables

Serves 4

45 ml/3 tbsp groundnut (peanut) oil

1 onion, sliced

5 ml/1 tsp salt

450 g/1 lb squid, cut into chunks

100 g/4 oz bamboo shoots, sliced

2 stalks celery, diagonally sliced

60 ml/4 tbsp chicken stock

5 ml/1 tsp sugar

100 g/4 oz mangetout (snow peas)

5 ml/ 1 tsp cornflour (cornstarch)

15 ml/1 tbsp water

Heat the oil and fry the onion and salt until lightly browned. Add the squid and fry until coated in oil. Add the bamboo shoots and celery and stir-fry for 3 minutes. Add the stock and sugar, bring to the boil, cover and simmer for 3 minutes until the vegetables are just tender. Stir in the mangetout. Mix the cornflour and water to a paste, stir into the pan and simmer, stirring, until the sauce thickens.

Braised Anise Beef

Serves 4

30 ml/2 tbsp groundnut (peanut) oil

450 g/1 lb chuck steak

1 clove garlic, crushed

45 ml/3 tbsp soy sauce

15 ml/1 tbsp water

15 ml/1 tbsp rice wine or dry sherry

5 ml/1 tsp salt

5 ml/1 tsp sugar

2 cloves star anise

Heat the oil and fry the beef until browned on all sides. Add the remaining ingredients, bring to a simmer, cover and simmer gently for about 45 minutes then turn the meat over, adding a little more water and soy sauce if the meat is drying. Simmer for a further 45 minutes until the meat is tender. Discard the star anise before serving.

Beef with Asparagus

Serves 4

450 g/1 lb rump steak, cubed

30 ml/2 tbsp soy sauce

30 ml/2 tbsp rice wine or dry sherry

45 ml/3 tbsp cornflour (cornstarch)

45 ml/3 tbsp groundnut (peanut) oil

5 ml/1 tsp salt

1 clove garlic, crushed

350 g/12 oz asparagus tips

120 ml/4 fl oz/¬Ω cup chicken stock

15 ml/1 tbsp soy sauce

Place the steak in a bowl. Mix together the soy sauce, wine or sherry and 30 ml/2 tbsp of cornflour, pour over the steak and stir well. Leave to marinate for 30 minutes. Heat the oil with the salt and garlic and fry until the garlic is lightly browned. Add the meat and marinade and stir-fry for 4 minutes. Add the asparagus and stir-fry gently for 2 minutes. Add the stock and soy sauce, bring to the boil and simmer, stirring for 3 minutes until the meat is cooked. Mix the remaining cornflour with a little more water or stock and stir it into the sauce. Simmer, stirring, for a few minutes until the sauce clears and thickens.

Beef with Bamboo Shoots

Serves 4

45 ml/3 tbsp groundnut (peanut) oil

1 clove garlic, crushed

1 spring onion (scallion), chopped

1 slice ginger root, minced

225 g/8 oz lean beef, cut into strips

100 g/4 oz bamboo shoots

45 ml/3 tbsp soy sauce

15 ml/1 tbsp rice wine or dry sherry

5 ml/1 tsp cornflour (cornstarch)

Heat the oil and fry the garlic, spring onion and ginger until lightly browned. Add the beef and stir-fry for 4 minutes until lightly browned. Add the bamboo shoots and stir-fry for 3 minutes. Add the soy sauce, wine or sherry and cornflour and stir-fry for 4 minutes.

Serves 4

225 g/8 oz lean beef

45 ml/3 tbsp groundnut (peanut) oil

1 slice ginger root, minced

100 g/4 oz bamboo shoots, sliced

100 g/4 oz mushrooms, sliced

45 ml/3 tbsp rice wine or dry sherry

5 ml/1 tsp sugar

10 ml/2 tsp soy sauce

salt and pepper

120 ml/4 fl oz/¬Ω cup beef stock

15 ml/1 tbsp cornflour (cornstarch)

30 ml/2 tbsp water

Slice the beef thinly against the grain. Heat the oil and stir-fry the ginger for a few seconds. Add the beef and stir-fry until just browned. Add the bamboo shoots and mushrooms and stir-fry for 1 minute. Add the wine or sherry, sugar and soy sauce and season with salt and pepper. Stir in the stock, bring to the boil, cover and simmer for 3 minutes. Mix the cornflour and water, stir it into the pan and simmer, stirring, until the sauce thickens.

Serves 4

45 ml/3 tbsp groundnut (peanut) oil

900 g/2 lb chuck steak

1 spring onion (scallion), sliced

1 clove garlic, minced

1 slice ginger root, minced

60 ml/4 tbsp soy sauce

30 ml/2 tbsp rice wine or dry sherry

5 ml/1 tsp sugar

5 ml/1 tsp salt

pinch of pepper

750 ml/1¬° pts/3 cups boiling water

Heat the oil and brown the beef quickly on all sides. Add the spring onion, garlic, ginger, soy sauce, wine or sherry, sugar, salt and pepper. Bring to the boil, stirring. Add the boiling water, bring back to the boil, stirring, then cover and simmer for about 2 hours until the beef is tender.

Beef with Bean Sprouts

Serves 4

450 g/1 lb lean beef, sliced

1 egg white

30 ml/2 tbsp groundnut (peanut) oil

15 ml/1 tbsp cornflour (cornstarch)

15 ml/1 tbsp soy sauce

100 g/4 oz bean sprouts

25 g/1 oz pickled cabbage, shredded

1 red chilli pepper, shredded

2 spring onions (scallions), shredded

2 slices ginger root, shredded

salt

5 ml/1 tsp oyster sauce

5 ml/1 tsp sesame oil

Mix the beef with the egg white, half the oil, the cornflour and soy sauce and leave to stand for 30 minutes. Blanch the bean sprouts in boiling water for about 8 minutes until almost tender then drain. Heat the remaining oil and stir-fry the beef until lightly browned then remove from the pan. Add the pickled cabbage, chilli pepper, ginger, salt, oyster sauce and sesame oil and stir-fry for 2 minutes. Add the bean sprouts and stir-fry for 2 minutes. Return the beef to the pan and stir-fry until well mixed and heated through. Serve at once.

Beef with Broccoli

Serves 4

450 g/1 lb rump steak, thinly sliced

30 ml/2 tbsp cornflour (cornstarch)

15 ml/1 tbsp rice wine or dry sherry

15 ml/1 tbsp soy sauce

30 ml/2 tbsp groundnut (peanut) oil

5 ml/1 tsp salt

1 clove garlic, crushed

225 g/8 oz broccoli florets

150 ml/¬° pt/generous ¬Ω cup beef stock

Place the steak in a bowl. Mix together 15 ml/1 tbsp of cornflour with the wine or sherry and soy sauce, stir into the meat and leave to marinate for 30 minutes. Heat the oil with the salt and garlic and fry until the garlic is lightly browned. Add the steak and marinade and stir-fry for 4 minutes. Add the broccoli and stir-fry for 3 minutes. Add the stock, bring to the boil, cover and simmer for 5 minutes until the broccoli is just tender but still crisp. Mix the remaining cornflour with a little water and stir it into the sauce. Simmer, stirring until the sauce clears and thickens.

Sesame Beef with Broccoli

Serves 4

150 g/5 oz lean beef, thinly sliced

2.5 ml/¬Ω tsp oyster sauce

5 ml/1 tsp cornflour (cornstarch)

5 ml/1 tsp white wine vinegar

60 ml/4 tbsp groundnut (peanut) oil

100 g/4 oz broccoli florets

5 ml/1 tsp fish sauce

2.5 ml/¬Ω tsp soy sauce

250 ml/8 fl oz/1 cup beef stock

30 ml/2 tbsp sesame seeds

Marinate the beef with the oyster sauce, 2.5 ml/¬Ω tsp of cornflour, 2.5 ml/¬Ω tsp of wine vinegar and 15 ml/ 1 tbsp of oil for 1 hour.

Meanwhile, heat 15 ml/1 tbsp of oil, add the broccoli, 2.5 ml/¬Ω tsp of fish sauce, the soy sauce and remaining wine vinegar and just cover with boiling water. Simmer for about 10 minutes until just tender.

Heat 30 ml/2 tbsp of oil in a separate pan and stir-fry the beef briefly until sealed. Add the stock, the remaining cornflour and fish sauce, bring to the boil, cover and simmer for about 10 minutes until the meat is tender. Drain the broccoli and arrange on a warmed serving plate. Top with the meat and sprinkle generously with sesame seeds.

Barbecued Beef

Serves 4

450 g/1 lb lean steak, sliced

60 ml/4 tbsp soy sauce

2 cloves garlic, crushed

5 ml/1 tsp salt

2.5 ml/¬Ω tsp freshly ground pepper

10 ml/2 tsp sugar

Mix together all the ingredients and leave to marinate for 3 hours. Barbecue or grill (broil) over a hot grill for about 5 minutes each side.

Cantonese Beef

Serves 4

30 ml/2 tbsp cornflour (cornstarch)

2 egg whites, beaten

450 g/1 lb steak, cut into strips

oil for deep-frying

4 stalks celery, sliced

2 onions, sliced

60 ml/4 tbsp water

20 ml/4 tsp salt

75 ml/5 tbsp soy sauce

60 ml/4 tbsp rice wine or dry sherry

30 ml/2 tbsp sugar

freshly ground pepper

Mix half the cornflour with the egg whites. Add the steak and mix to coat the beef in the batter. Heat the oil and deep-fry the steak until browned. Remove from the pan and drain on kitchen paper. Heat 15 ml/1 tbsp of oil and stir-fry the celery and onions for 3 minutes. Add the meat, water, salt, soy sauce, wine or sherry and sugar and season with pepper. Bring to the boil and simmer, stirring, until the sauce thickens.

Beef with Carrots

Serves 4

30 ml/2 tbsp groundnut (peanut) oil

450 g/1 lb lean beef, cubed

2 spring onions (scallions), sliced

2 cloves garlic, crushed

1 slice ginger root, minced

250 ml/8 fl oz/1 cup soy sauce

30 ml/2 tbsp rice wine or dry sherry

30 ml/2 tbsp brown sugar

5 ml/1 tsp salt

600 ml/1 pt/2¬Ω cups water

4 carrots, diagonally sliced

Heat the oil and fry the beef until lightly browned. Drain off the excess oil and add the spring onions, garlic, ginger and anise fry for 2 minutes. Add the soy sauce, wine or sherry, sugar and salt and mix together well. Add the water, bring to the boil, cover and simmer for 1 hour. Add the carrots, cover and simmer for a further 30 minutes. Remove the lid and simmer until the sauce has reduced.

Beef with Cashews

Serves 4

60 ml/4 tbsp groundnut (peanut) oil

450 g/1 lb rump steak, thinly sliced

8 spring onions (scallions), cut into chunks

2 cloves garlic, crushed

1 slice ginger root, chopped

75 g/3 oz/¬œ cup roasted cashews

120 ml/4 fl oz/¬Ω cup water

20 ml/4 tsp cornflour (cornstarch)

20 ml/4 tsp soy sauce

5 ml/1 tsp sesame oil

5 ml/1 tsp oyster sauce

5 ml/1 tsp chilli sauce

Heat half the oil and stir-fry the meat until lightly browned. Remove from the pan. Heat the remaining oil and stir-fry the spring onions, garlic, ginger and cashews for 1 minute. Return the meat to the pan. Mix together the remaining ingredients and stir the mixture into the pan. Bring to the boil and simmer, stirring, until the mixture thickens.

Slow Beef Casserole

Serves 4

30 ml/2 tbsp groundnut (peanut) oil

450 g/1 lb stewing beef, cubed

3 slices ginger root, minced

3 carrots, sliced

1 turnip, cubed

15 ml/1 tbsp black dates, stoned

15 ml/1 tbsp lotus seeds

30 ml/2 tbsp tomato pur√©e (paste)

10 ml/2 tbsp salt

900 ml/1¬Ω pts/3¬æ cups beef stock

250 ml/8 fl oz/1 cup rice wine or dry sherry

Heat the oil in a large flameproof casserole or pan and fry the beef until sealed on all sides.

Beef with Cauliflower

Serves 4

225 g/8 oz cauliflower florets

oil for deep-frying

225 g/8 oz beef, cut into strips

50 g/2 oz bamboo shoots, cut into strips

10 water chestnuts, cut into strips

120 ml/4 fl oz/¬Ω cup chicken stock

15 ml/1 tbsp soy sauce

15 ml/1 tbsp oyster sauce

15 ml/1 tbsp tomato pur√©e (paste)

15 ml/1 tbsp cornflour (cornstarch)

2.5 ml/¬Ω tsp sesame oil

Parboil the cauliflower for 2 minutes in boiling water then drain. Heat the oil and deep-fry the cauliflower until lightly browned. Remove and drain on kitchen paper. Reheat the oil and deep-fry the beef until lightly browned then remove and drain. Pour off all but 15 ml/1 tbsp of oil and stir-fry the bamboo shoots and water chestnuts for 2 minutes. Add the remaining ingredients, bring to the boil and simmer, stirring, until the sauce thickens. Return the beef and cauliflower to the pan and reheat gently. Serve at once.

Beef with Celery

Serves 4

100 g/4 oz celery, cut into strips

45 ml/3 tbsp groundnut (peanut) oil

2 spring onions (scallions), chopped

1 slice ginger root, minced

225 g/8 oz lean beef, cut into strips

30 ml/2 tbsp soy sauce

30 ml/2 tbsp rice wine or dry sherry

2.5 ml/¬Ω tsp sugar

2.5 ml/¬Ω tsp salt

Blanch the celery in boiling water for 1 minute then drain thoroughly. Heat the oil and fry the spring onions and ginger until lightly browned. Add the beef and stir-fry for 4 minutes. Add the celery and stir-fry for 2 minutes. Add the soy sauce, wine or sherry, sugar and salt and stir-fry for 3 minutes.

Deep-Fried Beef Slivers with Celery

Serves 4

30 ml/2 tbsp groundnut (peanut) oil

450 g/1 lb lean beef, cut into slivers

3 stalks celery, shredded

1 onion, shredded

1 spring onion (scallion), sliced

1 slice ginger root, minced

30 ml/2 tbsp soy sauce

15 ml/1 tbsp rice wine or dry sherry

2.5 ml/¬Ω tsp sugar

2.5 ml/¬Ω tsp salt

10 ml/2 tsp cornflour (cornstarch)

30 ml/2 tbsp water

Heat half the oil until very hot and fry the beef for 1 minute until just browned. Remove from the pan. Heat the remaining oil and fry the celery, onion, spring onion and ginger until slightly softened. Return the beef to the pan with the soy sauce, wine or sherry, sugar and salt, bring to the boil and stir-fry to heat through. Mix together the cornflour and water, stir into the pan and simmer until the sauce is thickened. Serve at once.

Serves 4

4 dried Chinese mushrooms

45 ml/3 tbsp groundnut (peanut) oil

2 cloves garlic, crushed

1 sliced ginger root, minced

5 ml/1 tsp salt

100 g/4 oz lean beef, cut into strips

100 g/4 oz chicken, cut into strips

2 carrots, cut into strips

2 stalks celery, cut into strips

4 spring onions (scallions), cut into strips

5 ml/1 tsp sugar

5 ml/1 tsp soy sauce

5 ml/1 tsp rice wine or dry sherry

45 ml/3 tbsp water

5 ml/1 tsp cornflour (cornstarch)

Soak the mushrooms in warm water for 30 minutes then drain. Discard the stalks and chop the caps. Heat the oil and fry the garlic, ginger and salt until lightly browned. Add the beef and chicken and fry until just beginning to brown. Add the celery, spring onions, sugar, soy sauce, wine or sherry and water and bring to the boil. Cover and simmer for about 15 minutes until the meat is tender. Mix the cornflour with a little water, stir it into the sauce and simmer, stirring, until the sauce thickens.

Chilli Beef

Serves 4

450 g/1 lb rump steak, cut into strips

45 ml/3 tbsp soy sauce

15 ml/1 tbsp rice wine or dry sherry

15 ml/1 tbsp brown sugar

15 ml/1 tbsp finely chopped ginger root

30 ml/2 tbsp groundnut (peanut) oil

50 g/2 oz bamboo shoots, cut into matchsticks

1 onion, cut into strips

1 stick celery, cut into matchsticks

2 red chilli peppers, seeded and cut into strips

120 ml/4 fl oz/¬Ω cup chicken stock

15 ml/1 tbsp cornflour (cornstarch)

Place the steak in a bowl. Mix together the soy sauce, wine or sherry, sugar and ginger and stir it into the steak. Leave to marinate for 1 hour. Remove the steak from the marinade. Heat half the oil and stir-fry the bamboo shoots, onion, celery and chilli for 3 minutes then remove them from the pan. Heat the remaining oil and stir-fry the steak for 3 minutes. Stir in the marinade, bring to the boil and add the fried vegetables. Simmer, stirring, for 2 minutes. Mix together the stock and cornflour and add it to the pan. Bring to the boil and simmer, stirring, until the sauce clears and thickens.

Serves 4

225 g/8 oz lean beef

30 ml/2 tbsp groundnut (peanut) oil

350 g/12 oz Chinese cabbage, shredded

120 ml/4 fl oz/¬Ω cup beef stock

salt and freshly ground pepper

10 ml/2 tsp cornflour (cornstarch)

30 ml/2 tbsp water

Slice the beef thinly against the grain. Heat the oil and stir-fry the beef until just browned. Add the Chinese cabbage and stir-fry until slightly softened. Add the stock, bring to the boil and season with salt and pepper. Cover and simmer for 4 minutes until the beef is tender. Mix the cornflour and water, stir it into the pan and simmer, stirring, until the sauce thickens.

Beef Chop Suey

Serves 4

3 stalks celery, sliced

100 g/4 oz bean sprouts

100 g/4 oz broccoli florets

60 ml/4 tbsp groundnut (peanut) oil

3 spring onions (scallions), chopped

2 cloves garlic, crushed

1 slice ginger root, chopped

225 g/8 oz lean beef, cut into strips

45 ml/3 tbsp soy sauce

15 ml/1 tbsp rice wine or dry sherry

5 ml/1 tsp salt

2.5 ml/¬Ω tsp sugar

freshly ground pepper

15 ml/1 tbsp cornflour (cornstarch)

Blanch the celery, bean sprouts and broccoli in boiling water for 2 minutes then drain and pat dry. Heat 45 ml/3 tbsp of oil and fry the spring onions, garlic and ginger until lightly browned. Add the beef and stir-fry for 4 minutes. Remove from the pan. Heat the remaining oil and stir-fry the vegetables for 3 minutes. Add the beef, soy sauce, wine or sherry, salt, sugar and a pinch of pepper and stir-fry for 2 minutes. Mix the cornflour with a little water, stir it into the pan and simmer, stirring, until the sauce clears and thickens.

Beef with Cucumber

Serves 4

450 g/1 lb rump steak, thinly sliced

45 ml/3 tbsp soy sauce

30 ml/2 tbsp cornflour (cornstarch)

60 ml/4 tbsp groundnut (peanut) oil

2 cucumbers, peeled, seeded and sliced

60 ml/4 tbsp chicken stock

30 ml/2 tbsp rice wine or dry sherry

salt and freshly ground pepper

Place the steak in a bowl. Mix together the soy sauce and cornflour and stir into the steak. Leave to marinate for 30 minutes. Heat half the oil and stir-fry the cucumbers for 3 minutes until opaque then remove them from the pan. Heat the remaining oil and stir-fry the steak until browned. Add the cucumbers and stir-fry for 2 minutes. Add the stock, wine or sherry and season with salt and pepper. Bring to the boil, cover and simmer for 3 minutes.

Beef Chow Mein

Serves 4

750 g/1 ¬Ω lb rump steak

2 onions

45 ml/3 tbsp soy sauce

45 ml/3 tbsp rice wine or dry sherry

15 ml/1 tbsp peanut butter

5 ml/1 tsp lemon juice

350 g/12 oz egg noodles

60 ml/4 tbsp groundnut (peanut) oil

175 ml/6 fl oz/¬œ cup chicken stock

15 ml/1 tbsp cornflour (cornstarch)

30 ml/2 tbsp oyster sauce

4 spring onions (scallions), chopped

3 stalks celery, sliced

100 g/4 oz mushrooms, sliced

1 green pepper, cut into strips

100 g/4 oz bean sprouts

Remove and discard the fat from the meat. Cut across the grain into thin slices. Cut the onions into wedges and separate the layers. Mix together 15 ml/1 tbsp of soy sauce with 15 ml/1 tbsp of wine or sherry, the peanut butter and lemon juice. Stir in the meat, cover and leave to stand for 1 hour. Cook the noodles in boiling water for about 5 minutes or until tender. Drain well. Heat 15 ml/1 tbsp of oil, add 15 ml/1 tbsp of soy sauce and the noodles and fry for 2 minutes until lightly browned. Transfer to a warmed serving plate.

Mix together the remaining soy sauce and wine or sherry with the stock, cornflour and oyster sauce. Heat 15 ml/1 tbsp of oil and stir-fry the onions for 1 minute. Add the celery, mushrooms, pepper and bean sprouts and stir-fry for 2 minutes. Remove from the wok. Heat the remaining oil and stir-fry the beef until browned. Add the stock mixture, bring to the boil, cover and simmer for 3 minutes. Return the vegetables to the wok and simmer, stirring, for about 4 minutes until hot. Spoon the mixture over the noodles and serve.

Serves 4

450 g/1 lb rump steak

10 ml/2 tsp cornflour (cornstarch)

10 ml/2 tsp salt

2.5 ml/¬Ω tsp freshly ground pepper

90 ml/6 tbsp groundnut (peanut) oil

1 onion, finely chopped

1 cucumber, peeled and sliced

120 ml/4 fl oz/¬Ω cup beef stock

Cut the steak into strips then into thin slices against the grain. Place in a bowl and stir in the cornflour, salt, pepper and half the oil. Leave to marinate for 30 minutes. Heat the remaining oil and fry the beef and onion until lightly browned. Add the cucumbers and stock, bring to the boil, cover and simmer for 5 minutes.

Baked Beef Curry

Serves 4

45 ml/3 tbsp butter

15 ml/1 tbsp curry powder

45 ml/3 tbsp plain (all-purpose) flour

375 ml/13 fl oz/1¬Ω cups milk

15 ml/1 tbsp soy sauce

salt and freshly ground pepper

450 g/1 lb cooked beef, chopped

100 g/4 oz peas

2 carrots, chopped

2 onions, chopped

225 g/8 oz cooked long-grain rice, hot

1 hard-boiled (hard-cooked) egg, sliced

Melt the butter, stir in the curry powder and flour and cook for 1 minute. Stir in the milk and soy sauce, bring to the boil and simmer, stirring, for 2 minutes. Season with salt and pepper. Add the beef, peas, carrots and onions and stir well to coat with the sauce. Stir in the rice then transfer the mixture to an ovenproof dish and bake in a preheated over at 200¬∞C/ 400¬∞F/gas mark 6 for 20 minutes until the vegetables are tender. Serve garnished with slices of hard-boiled egg.